CHEST RADIOLOGY COMPANION

Juan José Alva, M.D., FACP, ACAF

Ascension Thursday

05/17/07

CHEST RADIOLOGY COMPANION

ERIC J. STERN, M.D.
Associate Professor of Radiology and Medicine
Department of Radiology
University of Washington; and
Director, Thoracic Imaging
Department of Radiology
Harborview Medical Center
Seattle, Washington

CHARLES S. WHITE, M.D.
Associate Professor of Radiology and
Director, Thoracic Imaging
Department of Diagnostic Radiology
University of Maryland Medical School, Baltimore; and
University of Maryland Medical System, Baltimore,
Baltimore, Maryland

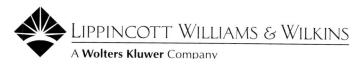

LIPPINCOTT WILLIAMS & WILKINS
A **Wolters Kluwer** Company
Philadelphia · Baltimore · New York · London
Buenos Aires · Hong Kong · Sydney · Tokyo

Acquisitions Editor: Joyce-Rachel John
Developmental Editor: Alexandra T. Anderson
Manufacturing Manager: Tim Reynolds
Production Manager: Liane Carita
Production Editor: Jeffrey Gruenglas
Cover Designer: Marsha Cohen
Indexer: Kathrin Unger
Compositor: Lippincott Williams & Wilkins Desktop Division
Printer: Maple-Vail

Printed in the United States of America

9 8 7 6 5 4 3 2

Library of Congress Cataloging-in-Publication Data
Stern, Eric J.
    Chest radiology companion / Eric J. Stern, Charles S. White.
        p.   cm.
    Includes bibliographical references and index.
    ISBN 0-397-51732-7
        1. Chest—Radiography.   2. Chest—Radiography—Case studies.
    I. White, Charles S.   II. Title.
        [DNLM: 1. Radiography, Thoracic.   WF 975 S839c 1999]
    RC941.S847 1999
    617.5′407572–dc21
    DNLM/DLC   98-46885
    for Library of Congress   CIP

To Karen–my beautiful, loving wife

E. J. S.

With love to my wife, Ellen, and to our children,
Billy, Rachel, and Danny

C. S. W.

Contents

Foreword

The interpretation of chest radiographs is a difficult task for a physician or radiologist at any level of training, but it can be particularly intimidating for a beginner. The accurate interpretation of plain films and chest CT scans may require a good eye, some experience with the range of appearances seen in normal subjects, and an ability to trace a path through a forest of anatomic detail without getting lost or misled. Unfortunately, these skills must be acquired through practice and through trial and error, and they are not easily learned by listening to a lecture or reading a book.

On the other hand, when interpreting radiographs, it is also important to have a set of rules to follow and rely upon when the going gets tough—rules about what is important to look for when a patient presents with cough or hemoptysis or shortness of breath; rules about what a lump or bump means or does not mean; and rules about what various diseases do and what they do not do. In this book Drs. Eric J. Stern and Charles S. White have attempted to provide some "rules to live by" to use when interpreting chest radiographs or CT scans. Within the pages of this book they provide a compendium of simple, easily digestible facts relating to specific chest diseases and diagnostic problems. They do so in a format they describe as being much like a slide lecture. Although this book will not make you a chest radiologist, it will, however, get you off to a good start.

W. Richard Webb, M.D.
University of California, San Francisco

Preface

The objective of this book is to serve as a practical, educational guide to interpreting the adult chest radiograph, one of the most commonly performed radiographic examinations and one of the most difficult to interpret.

It is our experience that no single approach to interpreting chest radiographs suffices. Although each chapter focuses primarily on differential diagnoses, the case presentation in this book offers a combination of approaches to image interpretation. When best suited, we use a basic pattern approach, an anatomic site of disease approach, or a disease process approach to image interpretation. When applicable, distinguishing features are highlighted.

The book is organized into five sections: 1) Methods; 2) The Lung; 3) The Mediastinum; 4) The Chest Wall, Pleura, and Diaphragm; and 5) Common Medical Problems. Each chapter is organized into appropriate and relatively common logical differential categories such as inflammatory processes, neoplastic processes, vascular processes, congenital processes, traumatic processes, etc., from the more common to the less common. By the very nature of categorizing, some topics can defy pigeonholing and may seem out of place, although we have tried to place such topics in the most logical of categories.

Given the bulleted lecture style, this book is practical and cannot be exhaustive or all inclusive. We cover the more common abnormalities encountered in the traditional hospital- and office-based radiology practice, as well as those topics considered radiology boards-oriented material. The cases selected are not meant to be all inclusive or pathognomonic, but representative. When appropriate, we hope to show a spectrum of possible presenting-disease features to give a more global understanding of the entity discussed.

We envision this book as a true companion, a working textbook that the reader can personalize and fine tune to his or her particular practice by adding additional bulleted notes to the appropriate pages.

The intended audience for this book is primarily radiology residents, but also includes medical students, pulmonary medicine trainees, and urgent/emergency department care providers (nurses, physician's assistants, etc.).

Section 1
METHODS

1 Chest Radiographic Fundamentals

Preliminary Evaluation

- Check the patient identity and date of the examination
- Orient the film on the viewbox
- Determine how the film was taken. Is it:
    Posteroanterior (PA) versus anteroposterior (AP)
    Upright versus supine versus decubitus
    Inspiration versus expiration
    Straight-on versus rotated
    Proper exposure
    Motion or other artifacts
- Check for comparison studies

Pattern of Study

The pattern order of study is less important than being diligent!
- Outside the patient
Look for any overlying artifacts that might obscure detail or be confused with an abnormality such as monitoring devices, clothes, hair, and so forth.
- Soft tissues
Check for changes in body habitus such as decreased muscle mass or subcutaneous fat, soft-tissue edema, overlying breasts or pectoral muscles, skin lesions.
- Bones
Check for normal development and mineralization, acute or healed fractures, degenerative changes, and dense or lytic abnormalities.
- Mediastinum
Check for any abnormal convexities or obscuration of normal structures such as the aorta and trachea. Always check for any deviation of midline structures such as the trachea or nasogastric tube. Recognize that the normal heart size can vary with age and depth of inspiration.
- Hila
Check for pulmonary vascular size, and masses or abnormal lobulation of hilar contours. The lateral radiograph is often the one most helpful in evaluating the hila. The avascular regions of the hila are the key to accurate evaluation. On the lateral radiograph these include:
1. Posterior wall of the bronchus intermedius
2. Left retrobronchial region
3. Region surrounding the right upper lobe bronchus
4. Inferior hilar window
- Lungs

Look for:

Size and distribution of the central airways and vessels
Volume loss by displacement of fissures, airways, and vessels
Silhouette sign, the loss of a normal profile (e.g., the right heart border)

Abnormal opacities or masses
Abnormal lucencies
Pleural margins
Lung symmetry

- Tubes and lines

Know the various monitoring devices, tubes, and lines that are commonly seen in your practice or hospital. Know their expected positions. Any device not in an expected position should be suspected as misplaced, the position checked clinically.

Repeat the above pattern of study for the lateral view.

Very important: Compare old films! They can be your best friend. Reviewing them may allow detection of a subtle new abnormality. More often it aids in specifying the cause of an abnormality (e.g., stable abnormality may indicate scar and no further workup, whereas a new abnormality may require further evaluation). This can save time, money, and patient anxiety.

2 Chest CT Protocols

It is easy to do the same protocol on every patient. However, it is often much better to tailor the chest computed tomography (CT) scan to the individual patient and patient problem. Here are some frequently used protocols, all differing in ways that optimize the CT evaluation of the patient's presenting clinical problem.

Thoracic Survey (Nonspiral)

Scan thickness and spacing: Apex 10 mm/10 mm; aortic arch to inferior pulmonary vein 5 mm/5 mm, base 10 mm/10 mm

Field of view: Smallest field of view capable of including entire chest and overlying soft tissues at its greatest width (generally 35–40 cm)

Range: Thoracic inlet to adrenals

Reconstruction algorithm: Mediastinum—standard
Lungs—bone/high resolution

Intravenous contrast: Yes (unless contraindicated by renal function, allergic history, department policy)

Rate: 2 mL/s × 40 seconds, 1 mL/s thereafter

Total volume: 150 mL

Scan delay: 12 seconds

Scan time: 1 second

Patient positioning: Supine

Respiration phase: End inspiratory

Filming parameter format: 12 on 1 (20 on 1, optional)

Window settings: Lung—W 1500 to 1800, L −700
Mediastinum—W 350, L 50
Liver—W 150, L 50

Special instructions: None

Thoracic Survey (Spiral) Also for rule out Metastasis

Table feed: 7 mm/s
Scan thickness: 7 mm
Pitch: 1:1
Field of view: Smallest capable of including bony thorax at its widest
Range: Thoracic inlet to adrenals
Reconstruction algorithm: Lung—bone/high spatial frequency
Mediastinum—standard
Intravenous (IV) contrast: None unless high suspicion for hilar metastasis
Patient position: Supine
Respiration phase: End inspiratory
Filming parameters: 12 on 1 (20 on 1, optional)

Window settings: Lung—W 1500 to 1800, L −700

Mediastinum—W 350, L 50

Liver—W 150, L 50

Special instructions: None

High Resolution CT for Interstitial Lung Disease

Scan thickness: 1 or 1.5 mm based on thinnest possible on scanner

Spacing: 10–20 mm

Range: Apex to base

Field of view: Select a field of view as small as possible to encompass the lungs.

Reconstruction algorithm: Bone/high spatial frequency

IV contrast: None

Scan time: As short as possible, 1 second

Patient positioning: Supine

Respiration phase: End inspiration

Filming parameters: Format: 6 on 1 (12 on 1, optional)

Window settings: Lung—W 1500, L −700

Mediastinum—W 350, L 50

Special instructions:

1. **Dependent density:** Turn patient prone and obtain scans of four sections of the lung bases (i.e., from carina inferiorly with intervals of 2 cm).
2. **Asbestosis workup:** Perform as #1 above
3. **R/O small airways disease:** Leave the patient supine and repeat examination as above at intervals of 2 cm in **expiration**. Film only inspiratory supine mediastinal windows (not prone, not expiratory). Film inspiratory and expiratory series in lung windows.

Emphysema Protocol

The emphysema protocol is used to evaluate for malignancy with the thoracic survey and for the emphysema with the high-resolution CT (HRCT).

Scan Thickness/Interval:

1. **Thoracic survey:** 10 mm/5 mm/10 mm as above
2. **HRCT:** 1 mm sections at 10 mm intervals inspiratory

1 mm sections at 20 mm intervals expiratory

Range: Thoracic survey: apex to adrenals

HRCT: Through lungs

Field of view: Smallest field of view capable of including all of chest and overlaying soft tissues at its greatest width (generally 35–40 cm)

Reconstruction algorithm: Lungs—Bone/high spatial frequency

Mediastinum—standard

IV Contrast: None

Patient positioning: Supine

Respiration phase: As above

Filming parameter format: Thoracic survey—12 on 1 (20 on 1, optional)
        HRCT: 6 on 1 (12 on 1, optional)

Window settings: Lung—W 1500, L −700 (for HRCT images)

    Mediastinum—W 350, L 50 (only film mediastinal
      windows of thoracic survey)

Solitary Pulmonary Nodule

Scan thickness: 3 mm (however, slice collimation should be no thicker than half the nodule diameter)

Table feed: 3 mm/s

Pitch: 1:1

Exposure duration: Single breathold through nodule (up to 30 seconds)

Range: Through nodule

Reconstruction algorithm: Bone/high spatial frequency algorithm

IV contrast: Following a noncontrast evaluation of the nodule, the section closest to the center will be selected. Omnipaque 300 (100 mL) at a rate of 2 mL/s will be administered and scanning at the level of the nodule will begin 30 seconds after the start of the injection.

Six single scans will be obtained at the level of the center of the nodule at 30-second intervals for the total elapsed time of 3 minutes. A thoracic survey will be performed after the 3 minutes of dynamic scanning.

Patient positioning: Supine

Respiration phase: End inspiratory

Filming parameters: Format: 12:1

Window settings: Lung—W 1800, L −700

    Mediastinum—W 350, L 50

Special instructions: Select center image on noncontrast image and perform pixel readout. Perform region of interest (ROI) measurements on each of the enhanced images.

R/O Thoracic Dissection

Scan thickness: 10 mm

Table feed: 10 mm/s

Range: Apex to diaphragm or through inferior most aspect of dissection if present

Reconstruction algorithm: Same as thoracic survey

IV contrast: 120 mL

Rate: 2 mL/s

Scan delay: 20 seconds

Scan time: 32 seconds

Patient positioning: Supine

Respiration phase: Inspiratory

Filming parameters: Same as thoracic survey

Special instructions: A few noncontrast scans may be obtained through the thoracic aorta. Supplement images with oblique/sagital/coronal reconstructions (4-mm interval reconstructions as needed)

Pulmonary CT Angiography

PART 1: Range: Spiral volumetric CT starting at the middle of the aortic arch and proceeding inferiorly for 10 cm. All patients should perform five deep breaths before suspending respiration.

    A. For patients who can suspend respiration for 20 seconds, feed with a collimation of 3 mm (pitch of 2). Images are reconstructed at 4-mm intervals (3 thick and 5 spacing = 1.7 pitch).

    B. For patients unable to suspend respiration well or on ventilator, feed with a collimation of 5 mm (pitch of 2). Images are reconstructed at 4-mm intervals.

Contrast: 120 mL at 3 mL/s

Scan delay: 20 second delay for normal hemodynamic status

Positioning: The arm receiving the contrast injection should be held above the patient's head to prevent venous compression at the thoracic inlet.

Additional instructions: Fill in areas not already covered after the initial run (i.e, apices to the level of the midaortic arch and the bases to the adrenals).

PART 2: [Optional for suspected chronic pulmonary embolism (PE)]: Screening unenhanced HRCT 1 mm/20 mm from apex to bases.

R/O Hemoptysis

The R/O hemoptysis protocol evaluates for two common causes of hemoptysis: malignancy with the contiguous 5 mm hilar portion and bronchiectasis with the HRCT.

Scan thickness: 1 or 1.5 mm at apex, 5 mm through hila, 1 or 1.5 mm through bases

Spacing: 10 mm at apex, 5 mm through hila, 10 mm through bases

Field of view: Smallest capable of spanning outer rib at widest portion of chest

Range: Thoracic inlet through lung bases

Reconstruction algorithm: Mediastinum—standard
                                Lungs—bone/high spatial frequency

IV contrast: Yes (unless contraindicated by renal function, allergy)

Rate: 2 mL/s × 40 seconds, 1 mL/s thereafter

Total volume: 150 mL

Scan delay: 12 seconds

Scan time: 1 second

Patient positioning: Supine

Respiration phase: End inspiratory

Filming parameter format: Lung—9 on 1

Mediastinum—12 on 1

Window settings: Lung—W 1800, L −700

Mediastinum—W 350, L 50

Special instructions: None

Lung Transplant

Scan thickness: 3 mm

Table feed: 5 mm/s (pitch of 1.7)

Reconstruction interval: 1 mm

Range: Apex to base

Reconstruction algorithm: Lung—bone

Mediastinum—standard

IV contrast: No

Scan time: 20-second breathold

Patient positioning: Supine

Respiration phase: End inspiratory 20-second breathold

Special instructions: Volumetric spiral acquisition starting 2 cm above the carina and scanning inferiorly for 10 cm in the z axis with 20-second breathold. Then fill in apex and base as needed. Reconstruct airway coronal in 1 mm intervals.

3 Dictations

Always answer the clinical question! For example, if the clinical problem is shortness of breath, cough, chest pain, and so forth, conclude your impression stating whether or are not specific features are found to explain the shortness of breath, cough, or chest pain. Also indicate pertinent negatives to the clinical question; for example, in patient's suspected of having a collagen vascular disease, note when no evidence is found of pleural effusion or thickening, no lung fibrosis, and so forth.

Speaking telegraphically, as though paying for every word, keeps reports short and concise.

Normal Adult Posteroanterior and Lateral Chest Radiograph

- The cardiomediastinal contour is normal. The lungs are clear. The bones and soft tissues are normal.

TELEGRAPHIC VERSION

Cardiomediastinal contour normal. Lungs clear. Bones and soft tissues normal.

Typical Intensive Care Unit (ICU) Supine Anteroposterior Chest Radiograph

The tubes and lines are in satisfactory and unaltered position. There is no change in the diffuse lung parenchymal opacities consistent with acute lung injury or acute respiratory distress syndrome (ARDS). There are no new focal abnormalities or barotrauma.

TELEGRAPHIC VERSION

- Tubes and lines in satisfactory and unaltered position. No change diffuse lung opacities consistent with acute lung injury/ARDS. No new focal lung disease or barotrauma.

ALTERNATE REPORT FOR AN ICU PATIENT, AS APPROPRIATE

- Tubes and lines in satisfactory and unaltered position. No change in mild lung edema and mild bibasilar atelectasis. No new focal disease.

Normal Chest Computed Tomography (CT) Scan

TECHNIQUE: SPIRAL CT

- Contiguous CT scans were obtained from the lung apices to the lung bases with 7 mm thick spiral sections, with intravenous contrast. Images were photographed at window and level settings suitable for viewing the lung parenchyma and soft-tissues.

TECHNIQUE: SPIRAL AND HIGH-RESOLUTION CT SCAN

Two series of images were obtained.

1. Contiguous CT scans were obtained from the lung apices to the lung bases with 7 mm thick spiral sections, with intravenous contrast.
2. 1.0 mm thick sections were obtained, with the patient supine, at 10 mm interval. Images were photographed at window and level settings suitable for viewing the lung parenchyma and soft tissues.

FINDINGS

The lungs, heart, and mediastinum are normal. The chest wall structures are normal. (Add appropriate pertinent negatives as per the clinical question.)

IMPRESSION

Normal chest CT scan.

TELEGRAPHIC VERSION

Lungs, heart, mediastinum normal. Chest wall structures normal.

4 Tube and Line Positions

Central Venous Catheters

KEY FACTS

CENTRAL VENOUS PRESSURE AND LARGE BORE CATHETERS:

- Central venous catheters are useful to infuse intravenous solutions or to measure central venous pressure. The ideal position for the tip of a central venous catheter is in the superior vena cava. This position is optimal for central venous pressure measurements.

- Catheter tip should be central to the venous valves that are found in the subclavian and internal jugular veins about 2 cm from their junction, at about the level of the first rib cartilage.

- On the lateral view, catheters inserted from the left side have an anterior convexity because of the anterior location of the left brachiocephalic vein. Catheters inserted from the right side descend in a straight course.

- Abnormal positioning of the central venous line occurs in up to 30% of patients. Commonly misplaced line locations are in the right atrium and ventricle, the inferior vena cava, the contralateral subclavian vein, internal jugular vein, and the azygos vein.

- Less commonly misplaced locations include a persistent left superior vena cava, the hepatic vein, internal mammary veins, and arterially in the aorta or subclavian artery.

- Catheters can be placed extravascularly, leading to mediastinal hemorrhage and extrapleural hematoma, or within the pleural space.

- Pneumothorax occurs more commonly with a subclavian approach.

SWAN-GANZ (PULMONARY ARTERY) CATHETERS

- Swan-Ganz (SG) catheters are placed in the pulmonary artery to measure pulmonary capillary wedge pressure.

- Catheter tip should be in the main left or right pulmonary arteries.

- On chest radiograph, the catheter tip is easily visible; SG balloon, at the tip, should not be inflated.

- If the catheter tip is too far distal, in the lung periphery, it can cause pulmonary infarction, which is recognized on chest radiography as a temporally-related wedge-shaped peripheral density, distal to the tip.

- SG catheter can rarely cause rupture of a pulmonary artery, leading to life-threatening hemoptysis.

- If pulmonary artery rupture is contained, a pseudoaneurysm can form.

- SG catheters can also cause arrhythmias because of irritation of the atrial or ventricular endocardium

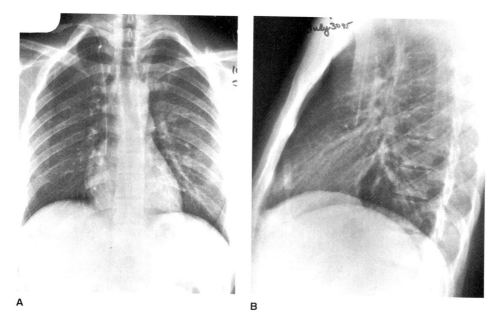

A   B

FIGURE 4-1   Posteroanterior **(A)** and lateral **(B)** chest radiographs show a well-positioned central venous catheter that has been inserted using a right internal jugular vein approach. Catheter tip is in the distal superior vena cava.

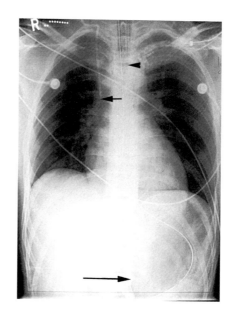

FIGURE 4-2

Posteroanterior chest radiograph shows a well-positioned central venous catheter *(short arrow)*, endotracheal tube *(arrowhead)*, and nasogastric tube *(long arrow)*.

(continued)

Central Venous Catheters (Continued)

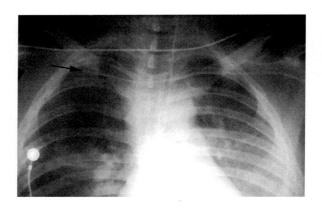

FIGURE 4-3

Anteroposterior chest radiograph shows a left subclavian venous catheter crossing inappropriately over to the right subclavian vein (*arrow*).

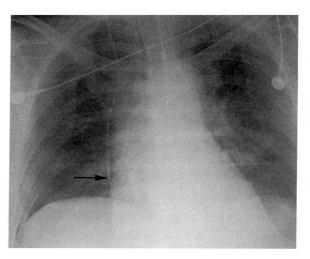

FIGURE 4-4

Anteroposterior chest radiograph shows a right subclavian venous catheter positioned lateral to the superior vena cava, in this case passing into the right internal mammary vein (*arrow*).

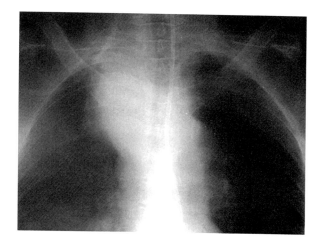

FIGURE 4-5

Anteroposterior chest radiograph shows a complication of central venous catheter placement, a large right-sided extrapleural hematoma. This occurred immediately after attempting a right subclavian line insertion, with inadvertent puncture of the subclavian artery.

Suggested Readings

Langston CS. The aberrant central venous catheter and its complications. *Radiology* 1971; 100:55–59.

McLoud TC, Putman CE. Radiology of the Swan-Ganz catheter and associated pulmonary complications. *Radiology* 1975;116:19–22.

Endotracheal Tube

KEY FACTS

- "The hose goes where the nose goes."—Michael "Benny" Benson. The endotracheal tube tip should be seen, optimally, ~4 cm above carina, ± 2 cm with head position. Therefore, always correlate chin level with the endotracheal tube tip.
- Unrecognized esophageal malposition is an uncommon ($\leq$ 1%) but potentially catastrophic complication of attempted endotracheal intubation
- Esophageal intubation can be diagnosed on chest radiographs by showing:
  1. Projection of any part of the endotracheal tube outside the tracheobronchial air column.
  2. An enlarged tracheal balloon cuff (transverse diameter > 2.8 cm).
  3. New extrapulmonary gas collections (marked gastric dilation, pneumoperitoneum, pneumomediastinum).
  4. Distal prolapse of the tracheal balloon (distal margin < 1.2 cm proximal to the endotracheal tube tip).
- Chest radiographs should be obtained routinely to verify correct endotracheal tube position.
- Gastric rupture and pneumoperitoneum following esophageal intubation and ventilation is rare, usually only occurring during cardiopulmonary resuscitation.
- If the endotracheal tube enters a bronchus (usually the right main bronchus because of the orientation of the airways), collapse of the contralateral lung usually occurs, and relatively quickly. The ipsilateral lung hyperinflates.

TRACHEOSTOMY TUBE

- Tracheostomy tube is inserted at the level of the third tracheal cartilage.
- Tip should be several centimeters above the carina.
- Tube should be approximately two thirds the width of the trachea and should project over the tracheal air column.
- Tracheostomy tube balloon should fill the trachea but not distend it.

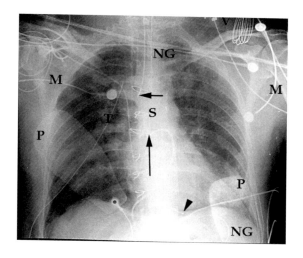

FIGURE 4-6

Anteroposterior supine chest radiograph shows a normally positioned endotracheal tube (*short arrow*), pulmonary artery catheter (*long arrow*), nasogastric tube (NG), femoral vein temporary pacing wire (arrowhead), and chest tube (T). Also note the overlying external pacer pads (P), sternal wires from a prior midline sternotomy (S), ventilator tubing (V), and cardiac monitoring wires (M).

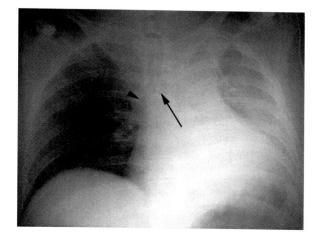

FIGURE 4-7

Anteroposterior chest radiograph shows accidental right mainstem intubation with subsequent hyperaeration of the right lung and near complete collapse of the left lung. The *long arrow* shows the tracheal carina and the *arrowhead* shows the endotracheal tube tip.

(continued)

Endotracheal Tube (Continued)

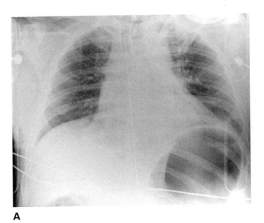 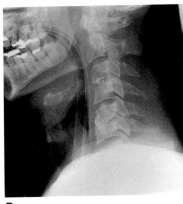

A   B

FIGURE 4-8   **(A)** Anteroposterior chest radiograph, as part of a trauma series, of a 52-year-old man shows gastric distention. The endotracheal tube was not seen. **(B)** Lateral cervical spine radiograph shows the esophageal intubation. Note the tracheal lumen anterior to the tube.

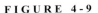

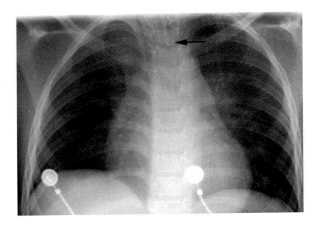

FIGURE 4-9

Anteroposterior radiograph, but with a slightly left anterior oblique (LAO) rotated chest view shows the endotracheal tube to the left of and obviously not within the trachea (*arrow*). This is an esophageal intubation.

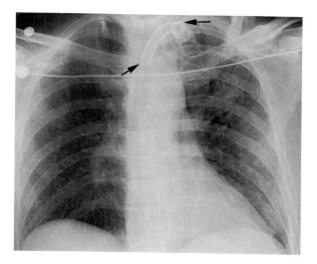

FIGURE 4-10
Anteroposterior chest radiograph shows a tracheostomy tube that is well positioned several centimeters above the carina (*arrows*).

Suggested Reading

Brunel W, Coleman DL, Schwartz DE, et al. Assessment of routine chest roentgenograms and the physical examination to confirm endotracheal tube position. *Chest* 1989;96: 1043–1045.

Enteral Tube Placement

KEY FACTS

- Feeding tubes (enteral tubes) and nasogastric tubes provide for instillation of peroral feedings or medications, or for gastric drainage.
- The tube is placed through the nose and courses through the esophagus to reach the stomach. The larger nasogastric tubes terminate in the stomach, whereas feeding tubes are usually placed in the duodenum.
- The entire length of many nasogastric tubes is radiopaque. The tip of the feeding tube is densely radiopaque and the remainder of the feeding tube is slightly radiopaque.
- On chest radiography, the tip of a correctly placed tube projects over the stomach or duodenum, as appropriate. The "appropriate position," is arguable, and differs from physician to physician, institution to institution, and patient to patient.
- Malposition of the feeding tube is the most common complication. The tip of the tube may be too proximal and lie in the esophagus. If the feeding tube is coiled in the hypopharynx, it may be largely or completely above the radiographic image.
- The feeding tube may inadvertently enter the trachea. On radiographs, it may be seen in the bronchi or lungs. Rarely, it can penetrate the pleura and cause a pneumothorax.
- Other complications include malposition in the mediastinum, abdomen, or cranium. Perforation of the esophagus can occur, but rarely.

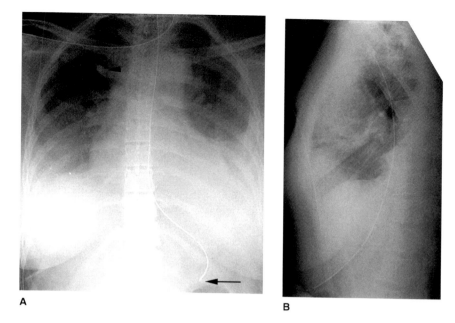

A   **B**

FIGURE 4-11   Posteroanterior **(A)** and lateral **(B)** chest radiographs show a normally positioned nasogastric tube, with the tip within the stomach (*arrow*). Note a normal azygous fissure (*arrowhead*), and bilateral pleural effusions.

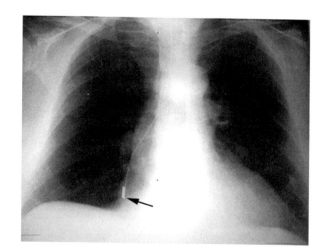

FIGURE 4-12

A weighted enteral feeding tube tip is seen within the medial basal segment of the right lower lobe (*arrow*).

Suggested Reading

Woodall BH, Winfield DF, Bissett GS II. Inadvertent tracheobronchial placement of feeding tubes. *Radiology* 1987;165:727–729.

Thoracostomy Tube

KEY FACTS

- Thoracostomy tubes are used to drain pleural collections of air or fluid.
- Tube should be placed anterosuperiorly for air collections and posteroinferiorly for fluid collections.
- Thoracostomy tubes that are placed in a fissure usually function adequately.
- The side hole of the chest tube should project inside the ribs.
- Malposition of the tube in the chest wall, mediastinum, or abdomen can be recognized on chest radiography, and lateral views are often valuable.
- Intraparenchymal placement of a chest tube is uncommon, and is most easily identified on computed tomography (CT) scan as a parenchymal hemorrhage with or without a large air leak.

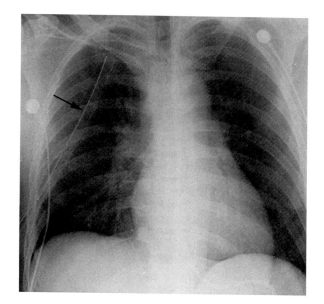

FIGURE 4-13

Anteroposterior chest radiograph shows a typical right thoracostomy tube that is well positioned in the right pleural space (*arrow*).

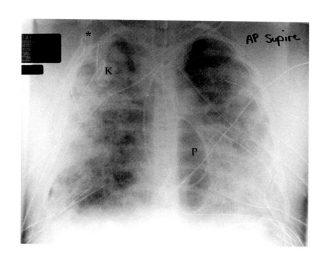

FIGURE 4-14

Anteroposterior chest radiograph from a 23-year-old woman with acute respiratory distress syndrome (ARDS) shows six right thoracostomy tubes and eight left thoracostomy tubes. One of the right thoracostomy tubes is extrathoracic (*) and one is kinked (*K*). A large pneumatocele (*P*), secondary to barotrauma, is seen within the left lung. This can be confused with a loculated pneumothorax.

Suggested Reading

Curtin JJ, Goodman LR, Quebbeman EJ, et al. Thoracostomy tubes after acute chest injury: relationship between location in a pleural fissure and function. *AJR* 1994;163:1339–1342.

Transvenous Pacemaker

KEY FACTS

- Two general types of pacemakers are available: permanent and temporary. They are used for a variety of cardiac arrhythmias.

- Pacemakers consist of a generator and a catheter that terminates in the right ventricle. Some pacemakers also have a catheter that paces the right atrium.

- The pacemaker wire can be placed in an abnormal position such as the coronary sinus or right ventricular outflow tract.

- Perforation of the right ventricular myocardium is rare, but it can lead to cardiac tamponade. On chest radiography, the perforated wire tip projects lateral to the heart on the frontal view or anterior to the epicardial fat stripe on the lateral view.

- Always check for pacemaker wire integrity.

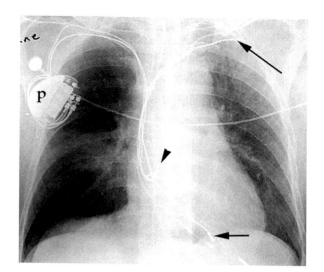

FIGURE 4-15

Posteroanterior chest radiograph shows a typical right-sided permanent dual lead pacemaker. The pacer tips are well positioned with one lead in the right atrium (*arrowhead*) and one in the right ventricle (*short arrow*). In this case, a prior left-sided pacemaker has been removed, with the old wires still in place (*long arrow*). Pulse generator (*p*).

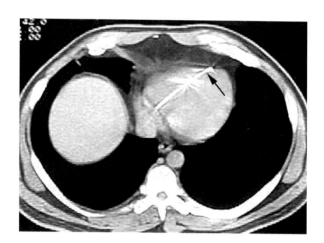

FIGURE 4-16

Computed tomography scan of the lower chest shows a metallic linear opacity within the right ventricle, as a normally positioned pacemaker lead.

Suggested Reading

Hall WM, Rosenbaum HB. The radiology of cardiac pacemakers. *Radiol Clin North Am* 1971;9:343–353.

Intra-Aortic Balloon Pump (IABP)

KEY FACTS

• The intra-aortic balloon pump is used to enhance cardiac output and increase perfusion to the coronary arteries in patients with cardiogenic shock. It consists of a fusiform inflatable balloon that measures approximately 26 cm.

• The IABP is inserted percutaneously using a femoral artery approach; it is advanced retrograde so that its tip lies immediately inferior to the origin of the left subclavian artery.

• The IABP deflates during systole to decrease afterload and inflates during diastole to facilitate coronary artery perfusion.

• If the tip is too proximal, the arch vessels may be occluded; if the tip is too distal the effectiveness of the IABP is reduced.

• On the chest radiograph, the IABP tip typically has a radiopaque marker, facilitating localization, although it can be difficult to recognize.

• If the radiograph is obtained during diastole, a tubular lucency of air is seen projecting over the descending thoracic aorta, which is caused by the helium gas within the inflated IABP.

• If a CT scan is obtained, air lucency may be detected within the aorta.

• Complications of IABP placement include malposition, aortic dissection or perforation, and femoral artery pseudoaneurysm.

Suggested Reading

Hyson EA, Ravin CE, Kelly MJ, et al. The intraaortic counterpulsation balloon: radiographic considerations. *AJR* 1977;128:915–918.

Section 2
THE LUNG

5 Lung Opacification—Diffuse

Pulmonary Edema

KEY FACTS

- Diffuse pulmonary opacities are often nonspecific. To formulate a simple but accurate differential diagnosis, think about what can make the lungs opaque: blood, pus, water, protein, and cells. The possible diagnoses will fall neatly in to place: pulmonary hemorrhage syndromes, pneumonias, pulmonary edemas, alveolar proteinosis, and certain malignancies such as bronchoalveolar carcinoma.

- It is obviously important to view the radiograph showing diffuse pulmonary opacities in light of prior examinations and in the clinical context. The clinical scenario for near drowning is certainly different from that of alveolar proteinosis or *Pneumocystis carinii* pneumonia, although the radiographs can appear similar.

Pulmonary edema can be classified into two types (see table below):

1. Increased capillary permeability (nonhydrostatic)
2. Elevated pulmonary venous pressure (hydrostatic).

The most important type of increased capillary permeability pulmonary edema is the acute respiratory distress syndrome (ARDS). ARDS is caused by diffuse alveolar damage, the severe end of the spectrum of diffuse lung injury, that occurs in multiple settings including sepsis, trauma, pneumonia, burns, and exposure to various toxins.

Hydrostatic pulmonary edema is often caused by congestive left-side heart failure, but can also be precipitated by fluid overload or renal failure.

The two types of pulmonary edema can often (but not always) be distinguished radiologically, particularly in early stages.

	HYDROSTATIC	NONHYDROSTATIC
Kerley's lines	Often present	Usually absent
Fissures	Thickened	Normal
Effusion	Frequent, especially on right	Usually absent or small
Pulmonary vessels	Redistribution	Normal
Bronchial walls	Cuffing	+/− Cuffing
Heart size	Enlarged	Normal
Distribution	Perhilar	Diffuse or peripheral
Vascular pedicle	Wide	Normal

A combination of the two edema types can occur, particularly once treatment is instituted, which can confound radiologic interpretation.

Atypical patterns of edema include unilateral or asymmetric edema. An example includes right upper lobe edema associated with acute mitral regurgitation, (see Chap. 6, p 84).

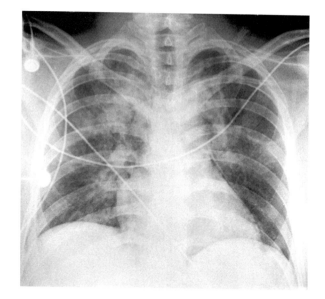

FIGURE 5-1

Anteroposterior chest radiograph of an 26-year-old-man who overdosed on intravenous heroin shows diffuse lung opacity consistent with pulmonary edema.

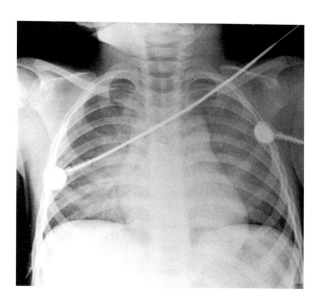

FIGURE 5-2

Anteroposterior chest radiograph of a 2-year-old-boy who had a chunk of a cheese sandwich lodged in his upper airway shows diffuse lung opacity consistent with negative pressure pulmonary edema.

(continued)

Pulmonary Edema (Continued)

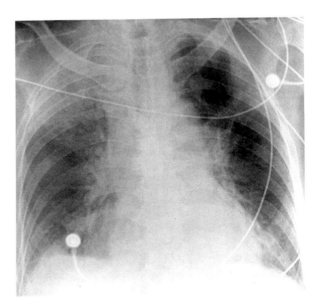

FIGURE 5-3
Anteroposterior chest radiograph of a 51-year-old-woman who suffered from smoke inhalation and severe airway injury shows diffuse lung opacity consistent with pulmonary edema.

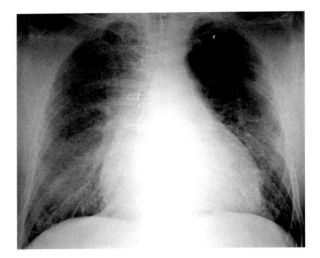

FIGURE 5-4
Anteroposterior chest radiograph of a 77-year-old-man with a long history of coronary artery disease shows diffuse lung opacity consistent with pulmonary edema caused by congestive left-sided heart failure. Note the prior midline sternotomy for coronary artery bypass grafting and the cardiomegaly.

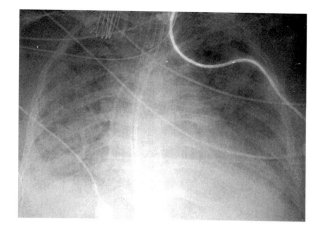

FIGURE 5-5

Anteroposterior chest radiograph of a 42-year-old-woman with ARDS shows diffuse lung opacity consistent with the diffuse alveolar damage and noncardiogenic edema of ARDS.

Suggested Reading

Putman CE. Cardiac and noncardiac edema: radiologic approach. In: Goodman LR, Putman CE, eds. Critical care imaging, 3rd ed. Philadelphia: WB Saunders, 1992.

Diffuse Pneumonia

K E Y   F A C T S

- Diffuse pyogenic pneumonia suggests an altered immune system, such as occurs in alcoholics or diabetics. Diffuse disease also suggests possible aspiration.

- Predisposing factors to aspiration include altered mental status, unconsciousness, general anesthesia, depressed gag reflex, swallowing disorders, and tracheal or esophageal intubation.

- Associated parapneumonic pleural effusions, which are common, often add to the overall diffuse lung opacification.

- Diffuse pneumonia can be caused by a multitude of organisms. Thus, the radiologic appearance is not specific and may be indistinguishable from pulmonary edema or pulmonary hemorrhage.

- A diffuse pneumonia that affects outpatients and usually resolves spontaneously is often caused by viral or Mycoplasmal infections. The chest radiographic findings of atypical pneumonias (e.g., *Mycoplasma pneumoniae*) may show fleeting unilateral or bilateral patchy segmental opacities or a diffuse interstitial (reticular) pattern.

- Acute pulmonary infection with the influenza virus results in a diffuse hemorrhagic pneumonia that can rapidly lead to respiratory insufficiency and death. The mortality rate in debilitated patients approaches 60% to 80%. Radiographic features range from mild interstitial prominence to diffuse alveolar damage leading to acute respiratory distress syndrome.

- Nosocomial infections, which are often diffuse, are typically caused by gram-negative bacteria such as *Pseudomonas* species.

- In the immunocompromised patient, diffuse pneumonia from bacterial, fungal, or *Pneumocystis* organisms are much more common than in the immunocompetent patient. In patients with acquired immune deficiency syndrome (AIDS) and *Pneumocystis* pneumonia, initial radiographs may show interstitial shadowing which progresses to widespread lung parenchymal opacity (see Chap. 6, p 70).

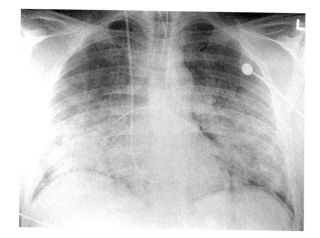

FIGURE 5-6

Anteroposterior chest radiograph of a 29-year-old-man with adenovirus pneumonia shows nonspecific diffuse lung opacity.

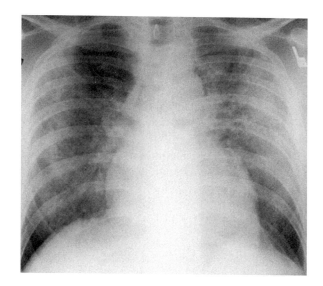

FIGURE 5-7

Posteroanterior chest radiograph of a 26-year-old-man with AIDS and *P. carinii* pneumonia shows typical bilateral perihilar lung opacities.

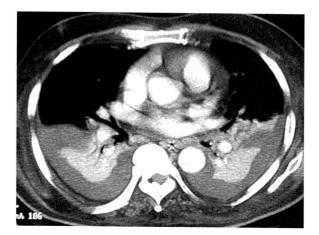

FIGURE 5-8

Chest computed tomography scan can often distinguish the different causes of diffuse lung opacification frequently seen on chest radiographs. Note the atelectasis of both lower lobes, surrounded by pleural effusions, both contributing to "whiteness" that would be seen on the radiograph.

Suggested Reading

Reyes MP. The aerobic gram-negative bacillary pneumonia. *Med Clin North Am* 1980;64:363.

Aspiration Pneumonia

KEY FACTS

- The clinical presentation of aspiration pneumonia depends on the material aspirated. Pneumonitis can be caused by aspiration of toxic fluids (e.g., gastric contents with ph < 2.5), bland fluids or particles (e.g., blood, water, food), or contaminated oral secretions.

- Toxic fluids cause a marked inflammatory reaction in the lungs. Chest radiographs show rapidly progressive patchy opacities in both lungs or predominantly the right lung base. Without development of secondary infection or ARDS, the radiograph appearance will clear within several days.

- Aspiration of bland material does not cause a chemical pneumonitis. The chest radiograph can be normal or have fleeting patchy opacities that clear with coughing or suctioning.

- Aspiration of oral anaerobic organisms found in the mouth (e.g., in those with bad dentition) can lead to aspiration pneumonia, necrotizing pneumonia, lung abscess, and empyema. Chest radiographs usually show opacities in gravity-dependent segments of lung.

- Predisposing factors to aspiration include altered mental status, unconsciousness, general anesthesia, depressed gag reflex, swallowing disorders, and tracheal or esophageal intubation.

- Endotracheal tubes with inflated cuffs do not afford complete protection against aspiration.

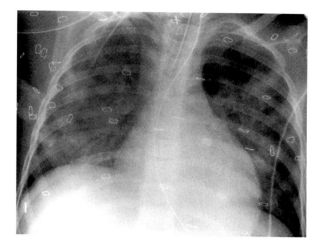

FIGURE 5-9

Anteroposterior chest radiograph of a 10-year-old-girl shows diffuse, patchy lung opacities with a perihilar distribution typical for the witnessed massive aspiration. Note the air-bronchograms in the right lung base. The staples are from skin grafting for burns.

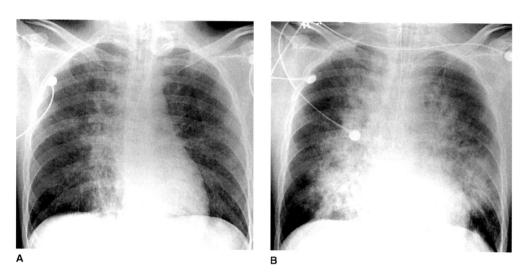

A

B

FIGURE 5-10   **(A)** Anteroposterior chest radiograph of a 37-year-old-man who had a massive aspiration of gastric contents shows bilateral perihilar lung opacity, right side > left side, typical of an aspiration. **(B)** The next day, the pneumonia is much worse, as is typical of many types of pneumonia. This eventually cleared over several weeks.

Suggested Reading

DePaso WJ. Aspiration pneumonia. *Clin Chest Med* 1991;12:269–284.

Pulmonary Hemorrhage

KEY FACTS

- Pulmonary hemorrhage can occur focally (e.g., bronchitis, bronchiectasis, tumor) or it can be diffuse.
- Diffuse pulmonary hemorrhage syndromes often coexist with renal disease. Anemia and hemoptysis are frequently present.
- Goodpasture's syndrome is caused by formation of antibodies to the antibasement membrane. It afflicts predominantly young white men, leading to diffuse pulmonary hemorrhage in combination with glomerulonephritis.
- Collagen vascular disease, especially systemic lupus erythematosus, is associated with pulmonary hemorrhage. It has also been reported with scleroderma, mixed connective tissue disease, and Henoch-Schönlein syndrome.
- In children, idiopathic pulmonary hemosiderosis is the most common cause of pulmonary hemorrhage. The bleeding is usually recurrent, with interval remissions, and ultimately results in pulmonary fibrosis.
- Anticoagulation and leukemia are uncommon causes of pulmonary hemorrhage.
- On chest radiographs, the appearance of pulmonary hemorrhage is nonspecific and consists of parenchymal opacity that can be patchy and nonuniform or can become confluent. Repetitive bleeding leads to the appearance septal lines from fibrosis.

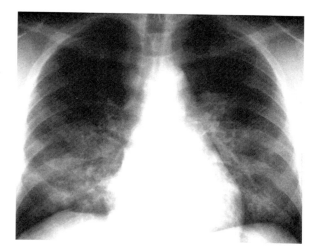

FIGURE 5-11

Posteroanterior and lateral chest radiographs of a 22-year-old-man with limited Goodpasture's syndrome shows nonspecific bilateral perihilar opacities as a result of pulmonary hemorrhage.

Suggested Reading

Albeda SM, Gefter WB, Epstein DM, et al. Diffuse pulmonary hemorrhage: a review and classification. *Radiology* 1985;154:289–297.

Pulmonary Alveolar Proteinosis

KEY FACTS

- Pulmonary alveolar proteinosis (PAP) is a disease of the lung that consists of the filling of the alveoli by a periodic acid Schiff (PAS)-positive proteinaceous material, rich in lipid, from uncertain causes. Features identical to those of PAP can occur after exposure to silica, fiberglass, volcanic dust, and aluminum dust.

- Chest radiographs typically show bilateral, patchy or diffuse, lung parenchymal opacification and, less commonly, an ill-defined nodular infiltrate, usually worse in the lung bases or perihilar regions. Cardiomegaly and pleural effusions are usually absent. Lymphadenopathy is rarely seen.

- The clinical and chest radiographic features of PAP can be indistinguishable from other common disorders such as pulmonary edema, pulmonary infection (viral, fungal, or *P. carinii*), neoplasms (in particular, bronchoalveolar carcinoma in a patient with few symptoms), pneumoconiosis, and even sarcoidosis.

- High resolution (HRCT) scanning of the chest, although not pathognomonic, can be particularly helpful in narrowing the differential diagnosis, often suggesting a specific diagnosis of PAP. HRCT scans show ground glass opacification and thickening of the intra and interlobular septa, with no architectural distortion, often in typical polygonal shapes called "crazy-paving," usually well demarcated from surrounding normal lung, creating a geographic pattern. Without clinical correlation, the HRCT scan pattern of crazy-paving is nonspecific, being reported in a variety of different diseases such as *P. carinii* pneumonia, lipoid pneumonia, ARDS, and sarcoidosis.

- Therapy for PAP is whole lung bronchoalveolar lavage, performed under general anesthesia. The prognosis is generally good with eventual quiescence of the disease in most patients.

- Superimposed confluent opacification, often as a new focal finding, can be caused by a secondary infection. Nocardia is frequently the cause of the superinfection in patients with alveolar proteinosis.

- Pulmonary alveolar proteinosis should be considered in the differential diagnoses of asymptomatic patients with chronic dyspnea on exertion who have diffuse lung opacities on chest radiographs.

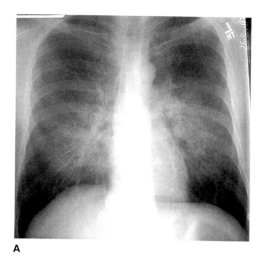

A

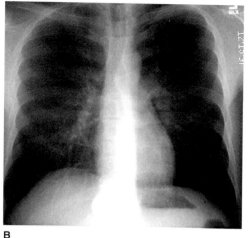

B

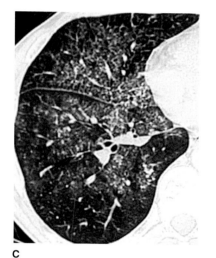

C

FIGURE 5-12

(A) Posteroanterior chest radiograph of a 37-year-old man with mild shortness of breath shows perihilar bilateral lung opacities. Eventual diagnosis was pulmonary alveolar proteinosis. **(B)** Posteroanterior chest radiograph obtained 2 months later, after therapy with bronchoalveolar lavage, shows a near normal radiograph. **(C)** HRCT scan from the same patient, obtained at the time of the initial chest radiograph shows the typical appearance for pulmonary alveolar proteinosis, with both ground glass opacification and thickening of the intra and interlobular septa, and no architectural distortion in polygonal shapes called "crazy-paving." Note the sharp demarcation from surrounding normal lung. (Case courtesy of S. Springmeyer, Seattle WA.)

Suggested Reading

Godwin JD, Müller NL, Takasugi JE. Pulmonary alveolar proteinosis: CT findings. *Radiology* 1988;169:609–613.

Near Drowning

KEY FACTS

- Two prominent components of near drowning are cerebral anoxia and pulmonary aspiration of water, the volume aspirated being more important than the nature of the fluid (fresh versus salt water).

- Radiographic assessment of near-drowning victims can vary greatly, ranging from a completely normal appearance to varying degrees of pulmonary edema.

- Important mechanisms of pulmonary edema formation appear to be loss of functional pulmonary surfactant, osmotically driven influx of plasma after salt water aspiration, and activation of inflammatory mediators with resultant diffuse alveolar damage and pulmonary capillary leakage.

- A 24 to 48 hour delay may occur before pulmonary edema develops or the edema may be present initially and resolve rapidly, even within hours.

- In most instances marked clearing of the lungs occurs within 3 to 5 days, with complete resolution of pulmonary edema within 7 to 10 days.

- In a near-drowning patient, scuba diving further increases the risks of developing lung barotrauma and decompression sickness.

- Mild decompression sickness (type I) symptoms relate to the formation of periarticular soft-tissue gas bubbles (the "bends").

- Severe decompression sickness (type II) results in inert molecular gas moving into the pulmonary or systemic arterial circulations ("gas embolism"), can result in pulmonary insufficiency (the "chokes") or central nervous signs and symptoms; severe decompression sickness, especially with cerebral gas embolism, always requires urgent hyperbaric therapy.

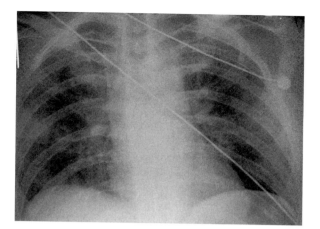

FIGURE 5-13

Anteroposterior chest radiograph of a 40-year-old-man who suffered near drowning while scuba diving at a depth of 40 feet shows diffuse parenchymal opacities consistent with pulmonary edema. Chest radiograph obtained 9 hours after (not shown), and after hyperbaric oxygen therapy, showed complete resolution of pulmonary edema.

Suggested Reading

Hunter TB, Whitehouse WM. Fresh-water near-drowning: radiological aspects. *Radiology* 1974;112:51–56.

Normal Exhalation

KEY FACTS

- Lung density on chest radiographs is inversely proportional to the amount of air in the lungs: A chest radiograph that is obtained in an expiratory phase appears substantially more dense than a radiograph exposed with full inspiration.

- Normal lung increases in density during exhalation in a consistent and linear manner related to the decrease in lung volume. By CT scanning, lung attenuation increases about 150 to 300 HU during exhalation, depending on the region of lung studied.

- A low lung volume radiograph can result from several different and important factors. The most common factor is a poor inspiratory effort, usually because of an inability to cooperate with breathing instructions. The patient may not speak the language in which the instructions are given, may have altered mental status, or may just be too weak to give much effort. All such factors yield the same finding of low lung volumes.

- A low lung volume radiograph can also be caused by intrinsic lung disease (e.g., interstitial pneumonitis), which can make the lungs less compliant or "stiffer." This will give the patient a sensation of dyspnea, as well as make it harder for the patient to take as deep a breath as would otherwise be possible. In this situation, the lungs appear more dense than normal but it is often not possible to distinguish true mild diffuse interstitial lung disease from a poor inspiratory result.

- Almost all chest radiographs are and should be obtained at full suspended inspiration. If the patient cannot take a full breath and hold it, the normal increased density of an expiratory radiograph may be judged to be pathologic. The increased lung density can be misinterpreted as diffuse lung disease, particularly pulmonary edema or diffuse pneumonia.

- Expiratory radiography can be used in tandem with inspiratory radiography to diagnose air trapping as can occur with foreign body inhalation. In the presence of an obstructing foreign body, air trapping prevents egress of air; there is little or no increase in lung density during the expiratory phase.

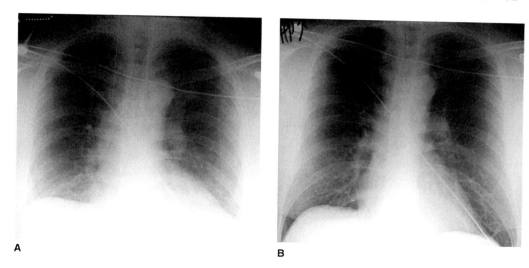

A   **B**

FIGURE 5-14. **(A)** Anteroposterior chest radiograph of a 50-year-old-man with severe chest pain shows a nonspecific diffuse increase in lung opacity, suggestive of pulmonary edema. **(B)** A repeat chest radiograph taken of the same man just moments later, but with greater inhalation, shows no evidence of lung disease.

Suggested Reading

Webb WR, Stern EJ, Kanth N, et al. Dynamic pulmonary CT: findings in healthy adult men. *Radiology* 1993;186:117–124.

6 Lung Opacification—Focal

Bacterial Pneumonia

KEY FACTS

- Radiographic patterns of pneumonia can be classified as lobar pneumonia, bronchopneumonia, and interstitial pneumonia.

- Lobar pneumonia is caused by interalveolar spread of exudate through pores of Kohn and canals of Lambert. It is delimited by fissures. The prototype organism is *Streptococcus pneumoniae*, but lobar pneumonia can be caused by many different bacteria.

- Bronchopneumonia disseminates through conducting airways and it is more diffuse and patchy than lobar pneumonia. The prototype organism is *Staphylococcus aureus*.

- Interstitial pneumonia extends along septal margins of lung and demonstrates a reticular appearance. Atypical and viral pneumonias often show this pattern.

- The diagnosis of pneumonia is based on clinical evaluation, plus appropriate radiographic and laboratory studies.

- To limit differential diagnoses, pulmonary infections should be thought of as occurring in various clinical subsets: community acquired, nosocomial, and immunocompromised patient populations. Correlate the clinical information with the dominant chest radiographic features (e.g., unilateral lobar opacification, diffuse interstitial infiltrates, adenopathy, and so forth) to limit the differential diagnosis of possible causative pathogens.

- The most common community-acquired pneumonias are
Gram positive:
Pneumococcal pneumonia
Staphylococcus aureus pneumonia (e.g., postinfluenza, intravenous drug users)
Gram negative:
Klebsiella pneumoniae (especially in alcoholics)
Pseudomonas pneumoniae (nosocomial)
Haemophilus pneumonia (especially in chronic lung disease)
Also:
Legionnaires' disease
Mycoplasma pneumoniae

- Typically appear radiographically as near-lobar or lobar opacification, usually with air-bronchograms.

- Multilobar opacification suggests an altered immune system, such as occurs in alcoholics or diabetics. Multilobar disease also suggests possible aspiration.

- Associated parapneumonic pleural effusions are common. Development of frank empyema, which is less common, is not distinguishable radiographically.

- Bronchopneumonia, which disseminates through conducting airways, is more diffuse and patchy than lobar pneumonia. The prototype organism is *S. aureus*.

- Interstitial pneumonia extends along septal margins of lung and demonstrates a reticular appearance. Atypical and viral pneumonias often show this pattern.

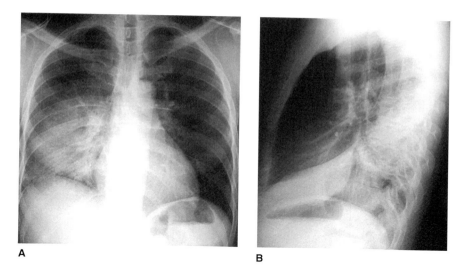

F I G U R E 6 - 1   Posteroanterior **(A)** and lateral **(B)** chest radiograph of a 34-year-old man with fever and productive cough shows a dense opacity in the right lower lobe, typical of lobar pneumonia.

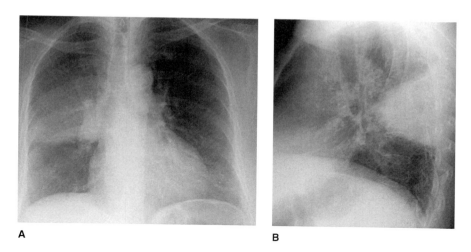

F I G U R E 6 - 2   Posteroanterior **(A)** and lateral **(B)** chest radiograph of a 29-year-old man with fever and productive cough shows a dense opacity in the superior segment of the right lower lobe, typical of a segmental pneumonia.

(continued)

Bacterial Pneumonia *(Continued)*

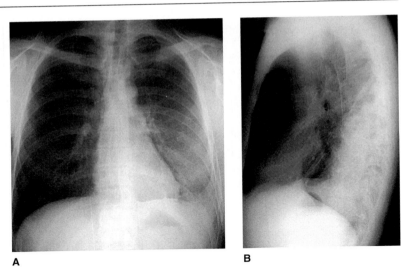

A   B

FIGURE 6-3   Posteroanterior **(A)** and lateral **(B)** chest radiograph of a 33-year-old man with new onset fever and productive cough shows a dense opacity with a left lower lobe distribution, typical of a lobar pneumonia.

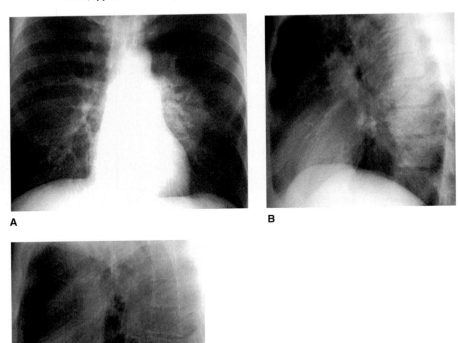

A   B

C

FIGURE 6-4

Posteroanterior **(A)** and lateral **(B)** chest radiograph of a 43-year-old-man shows a wedge-shaped opacity in the superior segment of the left lower lobe, typical for a bacterial pneumonia. Follow-up lateral radiograph several weeks later shows the pneumonia has cleared.

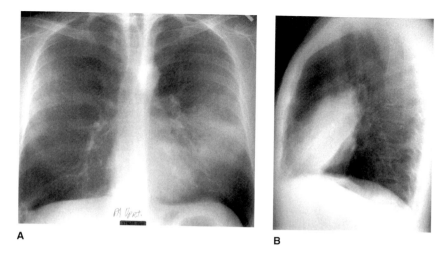

FIGURE 6-5   Posteroanterior (**A**) and lateral (**B**) chest radiograph of a 51-year-old-man shows a wedge-shaped opacity in the lingula, typical of a bacterial pneumonia.

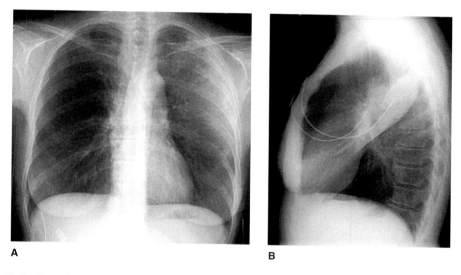

FIGURE 6-6   Posteroanterior (**A**) and lateral (**B**) chest radiograph of a 34-year-old-woman shows a wedge-shaped opacity in the left upper lobe, typical for a bacterial pneumonia.

(continued)

Bacterial Pneumonia *(Continued)*

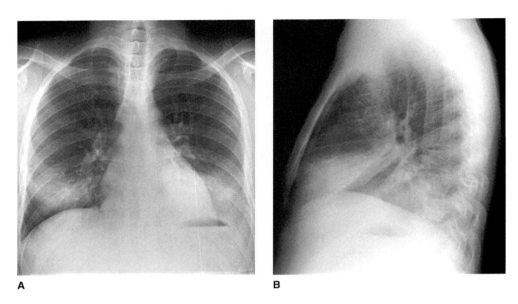

A   B

F I G U R E   6 - 7   Posteroanterior **(A)** and lateral **(B)** chest radiograph of a 47-year-old-man shows opacities in the right middle lobe and the left lower lobe, typical for a bacterial pneumonia.

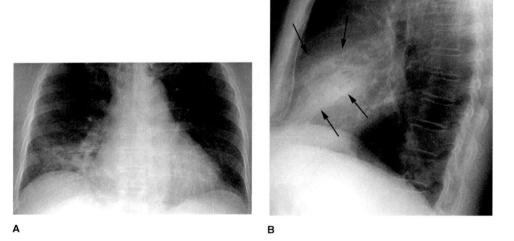

A   B

F I G U R E   6 - 8   Posteroanterior **(A)** and lateral **(B)** chest radiograph of a 54-year-old-man shows opacity in the right middle lobe, again typical for a bacterial pneumonia. These pneumonias are often best seen on the lateral view *(arrows)*.

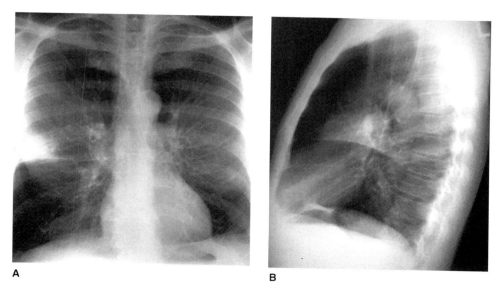

FIGURE 6-9   Posteroanterior **(A)** and lateral **(B)** chest radiograph of a 29-year-old-man shows a wedge-shaped opacity in the axillary subsegment of the right upper lobe, typical for a pneumonia.

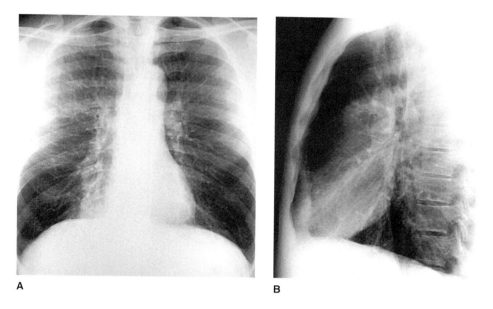

FIGURE 6-10   Posteroanterior **(A)** and lateral **(B)** chest radiograph of a 46-year-old-man shows a wedge-shaped opacity in the medial basal segment of the right lower lobe, typical for a pneumonia. This case is of additional interest because the pneumonia is confined to the medial basal segment of the right lower lobe by an inferior accessory fissure.

Suggested Reading

Mittl RL, Schwab RJ, Duchin JS, et al. Radiographic resolution of community-acquired pneumonia. *Am J Respir Crit Care Med* 1994;149:630–635.

Atypical Pneumonia

KEY FACTS

- An atypical pneumonia presents clinically as a systemic infection rather than a typical community-acquired lobar pneumonia, especially considering the many possible extrapulmonary manifestations.

- *Mycoplasma* pneumonia is a common community-acquired pneumonia, often classified as an atypical pneumonia that produce a wide range of upper respiratory symptoms, from acute pneumonias in otherwise healthy adults to rare reports of acute respiratory distress syndrome (ARDS) to otitis or sinusitis in children.

- Most cases of *Mycoplasma* pneumonia (up to 90%) are probably not detected clinically and, therefore, its true incidence is unknown.

- The most frequent extrapulmonary manifestations of *Mycoplasma* pneumonia are arthralgias and myalgias. Other less common manifestations involve hematologic, dermatologic, cardiac, neurologic, gastrointestinal, and hematologic organ systems; they include autoimmune hemolytic anemia, hepatitis, erythema nodosum, myocarditis, and meningitis.

- The chest radiographic findings of atypical pneumonia in the adult are nonspecific and may show fleeting unilateral or bilateral patchy segmental opacities or a diffuse interstitial (reticular) pattern not unlike that of a viral pneumonia.

- Other atypical pneumonias with similar radiographic features include infections by *Chlamydia psittaci* (psittacosis or ornithosis) and *Coxiella burnetti* (Q fever).

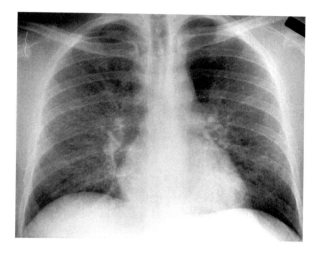

FIGURE 6-11

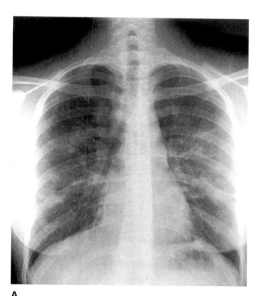

A

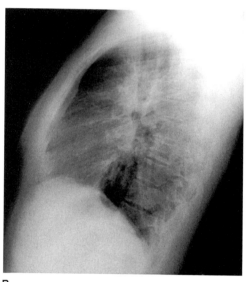

B

FIGURES 6-11 and 6-12   Posteroanterior chest radiographs (**6-11** and **6-12A**) and lateral (**6-12B**) of two patients with acute onset of myalgias, cough, and fever show coarse, diffuse interstitial abnormalities consistent with an atypical community-acquired pneumonia, in these cases caused by *M. pneumoniae.*

Suggested Reading

Martin RE, Bates JH. Atypical pneumonia. *Infect Dis Clin North Am* 1991;5:585–601.

Viral Pneumonia

KEY FACTS

- The most common viruses that cause pulmonary infections are:
  Adenovirus
  Herpes virus (varicella)
  Influenza virus
  Respiratory syncytial virus
  Measles
  Parainfluenza

- Adenoviral pneumonia is rare and occurs sporadically. It may be mild or severe and it is usually accompanied by upper respiratory symptoms. Early chest radiographic findings show a fine reticular infiltrate, corresponding to interstitial inflammation, seldom involving more than a single lower lobe. The inflammation may, however, produce patchy air space opacification. As the pneumonia resolves, clinically, persistent interstitial infiltrate may exist.

- Varicella pneumonia is an acute chickenpox pneumonia that usually occurs in adults who have severe cutaneous disease. Clinical and radiographic features of varicella pneumonia develop 2 to 5 days after the skin lesions. The chest radiograph most commonly shows diffuse small nodular opacities with a peribronchovascular distribution, probably reflecting contiguous spread from tracheobronchitis. The nodules are ill-defined and usually less than 5 mm in diameter. The radiographic appearance can be similar to other interstitial processes (e.g., sarcoidosis, miliary tuberculosis, or lymphangitic carcinomatosis); but, in light of these various clinical presentations, a diagnostic dilemma does not usually occur. Chest radiographic clearing may take from 10 days to several months, or even years. Rarely, however, the nodules can calcify (less than 2%).

- Acute pulmonary infection with the influenza virus results in a diffuse hemorrhagic pneumonia that can rapidly lead to respiratory insufficiency and death. The mortality rate in debilitated patients approaches 60% to 80%. Overall, acute primary influenza pneumonia is rarely seen in more than 1% of infected individuals. Radiographic features range from mild interstitial prominence to diffuse alveolar damage leading to acute respiratory distress syndrome. Cavity formation suggests bacterial superinfection.

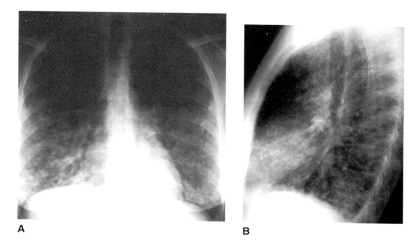

A   B

FIGURE 6-13   Posteroanterior **(A)** and lateral **(B)** chest radiograph of a 29-year-old woman with cutaneous chickenpox (varicella), fever, and cough shows diffuse coarse interstitial opacities with a somewhat basilar predominance consistent with varicella pneumonia.

Suggested Reading
Greenberg SB. Viral pneumonia. *Infect Dis Clin North Am* 1991;5:603–621.

Mycobacterial Pneumonia

KEY FACTS

- The incidence of active tuberculosis in the United States has steadily declined over the last 40 years, mostly because of improved detection, public health measures, and adequate antibiotic regimens. However, the incidence has increased in recent years, particularly among indigent minority groups living in urban centers. This partly relates to the prevalence of human immunodeficiency virus (HIV) infection in these groups.

PRIMARY TUBERCULOSIS

- Primary tuberculosis is usually thought of as an infection of the extreme age groups, the pediatric or elderly. It is now also seen in young adults, especially HIV-infected individuals.
- On inhalation, the *Mycobacterium tuberculosis* organism initially infects a gravity-dependent area of the lung. Lymphatic invasion leads to hilar lymph node involvement, followed by hematogenous dissemination throughout the body where the organisms can remain dormant for decades and serve as a focus for potential reactivation, especially the lung apices.
- The chest radiograph shows a homogeneous opacity, without cavitation, which can involve either the upper or lower lobes in combination with mediastinal/hilar lymph node enlargement. This adenopathy can be the striking finding in children and clearly differentiates primary from secondary tuberculosis, in patients with a normal immune system.
- Subsequent chest radiographs may show calcified or noncalcified pulmonary (Ghon lesion) and hilar lymph node (Ranke nodes) granulomas, which in combination are referred to as the "primary complex."
- No clinical evidence of disease is found in 95% of individuals with primary pulmonary tuberculosis. Symptoms, when present, are usually mild and nonspecific, resolving completely without specific therapy.
- Other less common presentations of primary tuberculosis include tracheobronchial compression of bronchi by enlarged lymph nodes and large unilateral pleural effusions.
- In a small percentage of cases, adequate cell-mediated immunity does not develop, and progressive and symptomatic primary pulmonary disease will occur.

SECONDARY, POSTPRIMARY, OR REACTIVATION TUBERCULOSIS

- Most cases present either as a result of an abnormal screening chest radiograph, or from vague complaints of nonspecific constitutional symptoms and chronic cough.
- Reactivation tuberculosis tends to involve the apical or posterior segments of the upper lobes.
- Protean clinical and chest radiographic manifestations may be seen with reactivation tuberculosis, with affected individuals often showing one or more abnormalities. The most common is the typical apical fibrocavitary lesions. Caseous necrosis and cavitation allow the endobronchial

dissemination of organisms, or bronchogenic spread, which is suggestive of communicability. Hematogenous dissemination of organisms occurs with an impaired immune system leading to miliary tuberculosis, with innumerable tiny (< 3 mm) discrete nodules scattered widely and rather uniformly (in a hematogenous distribution) throughout the lungs. Tuberculous pleurisy, empyema, or bronchopleural fistula can develop as a result of infection in the pleural space. When healed, this results in extensive pleural fibrosis and calcification. The airways can be involved in several ways. Endobronchial occlusion and air trapping may result from an endobronchial granuloma or eroding hilar lymph node. Postinflammatory bronchiectasis may occur; seen most commonly in the right middle lobe, it is one of the causes of "right middle lobe syndrome." A mycetoma, or fungus ball, most commonly *Aspergillus* species, may form in tuberculous cavities. The dreaded complication of a mycetoma formation within a tuberculous cavity is erosion of a pulmonary artery (Rasmussen's aneurysm) causing life-threatening hemoptysis.

- Mycobacterial organisms other than tuberculosis are also pathogenic, although much less common, often occurring in immunocompromised hosts; for example, *M. avium-intracellulare*, *M. kansasii*, and *M. gordonii*.

- Infectious activity is difficult to assess radiographically. Avoid descriptive expressions such as old granulomatous disease or "OGD." Unless evidence suggestive of endobronchial spread of organisms (apical fibrocavitary disease with bilateral or contralateral perihilar fluffy opacities) exists, it is better to state that chest radiographic evidence indicates a prior granulomatous infection of indeterminate activity.

- Comparison films are essential in determining infectious activity. Computed tomography (CT) scanning can detect unsuspected activity, often distinguishing a quiescent prior infection from new disease. The CT scan findings of infectious activity are small, ill-defined nodules with a bronchovascular distribution ("tree-in-bud") as evidence of active endobronchial disease and, therefore, of a potential public health hazard. This finding is also seen in many other abnormalities, most of which are infectious or granulomatous bronchiolar processes.

(continued)

Mycobacterial Pneumonia *(Continued)*

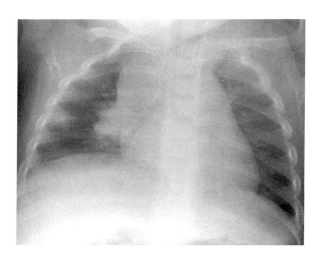

FIGURE 6-14

Anteroposterior chest radiograph of a 2-year-old-child shows a small peripheral, ill-defined opacity in the right midlung and enlargement of the right hilum caused by adenopathy. The superior mediastinal widening is more likely caused by a normal thymus. This is a classic presentation of primary tuberculous infection.

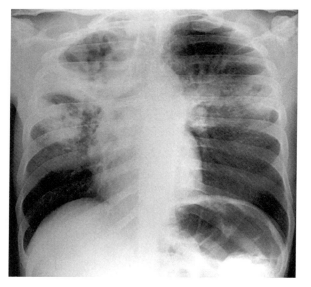

FIGURE 6-15

Anteroposterior chest radiograph of a 43-year-old man with several month's history of fever, cough, night sweats, and weight loss shows typical features of reactivation tuberculosis with endobronchial spread. Note the right upper lobe thick-walled cavitation with bilateral perihilar fluffy parenchymal opacities (the endobronchial spread). This appearance should alert the radiologist and clinician to the true public health hazard that this patient represents. This patient was isolated immediately and found to have florid amounts of *Mycobacterium* organisms in his sputum.

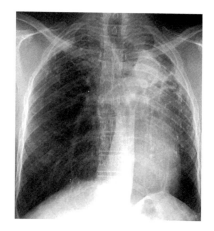

FIGURE 6-16

Posteroanterior chest radiograph of a 57-year-old man with a history of adequately treated tuberculosis contrasts with the case illustrated in Figure 6-15. Note the extensive scarring in the left upper lobe with volume loss and retraction of the trachea and left hilum. This radiographic appearance should be viewed as indeterminate for tuberculous activity and compared with prior radiographs to determine stability.

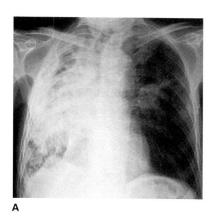

A

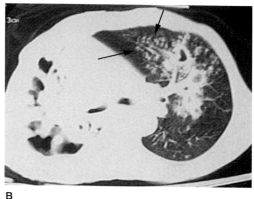

B

FIGURE 6-17 (A) Posteroanterior chest radiograph of a 63-year-old man with a floridly sputum-positive tuberculosis shows extensive cavitary right lung destruction and ill-defined nodular opacities in the left midlung. These nodular opacities are strongly suggestive of endobronchial spread of tuberculosis, a sign of an actively infectious individual. (B) CT scan shows the cavitary disease and the tree-in-bud (*arrows*) pattern of endobronchial spread of disease to better advantage.

Suggested Reading

Buckner CB, Walker CW. Radiologic manifestations of adult tuberculosis. *J Thorac Imaging* 1990;5:28–37.

Fungal Pneumonia

KEY FACTS

- Fungal infections of the lung are seen in both healthy and immuncompromised individuals.
- The most prevalent pulmonary fungal infections are histoplasmosis, coccidioidomycosis, and blastomycosis.
- When the clinical and radiographic diagnosis suggests tuberculosis, the differential diagnosis should include histoplasmosis, coccidioidomycosis, and blastomycosis. The radiographic features of fungal pneumonias are usually nonspecific, although often they take a more indolent time course than bacterial pneumonias.
- Patient demographics are often helpful in narrowing the differential diagnosis. Blastomycosis is seen commonly in the southeastern United States. Histoplasmosis is endemic in the Mississippi and Ohio river valleys. Coccidioidomycosis is endemic in the southwestern United States and the central valley of California.
- (See Chap. 8 for more on fungal infections.)

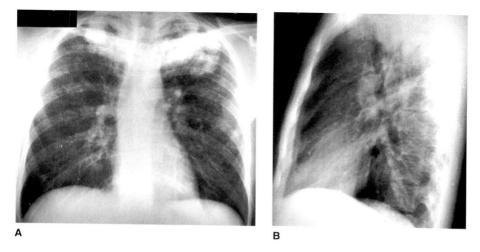

A   **B**

FIGURE 6-18   Posteroanterior **(A)** and lateral **(B)** chest radiographs of a 37-year-old immunocompromised man with cryptococcal pneumonia shows nonspecific, bilateral upper
lobe opacities.

Suggested Reading

Haque AK. Pathology of common pulmonary fungal infections. *J Thorac Imaging* 1992;
7:1–11.

Pneumonia in the Immunocompromised Patient (AIDS)

KEY FACTS

- Patients with acquired immune deficiency syndrome (AIDS) can and do still get typical community-acquired, bacterial pneumonia.

- *Pneumocystis carinii*, which is the agent that most commonly causes pneumonia in this population, is seen in up to two thirds of presenting cases. Typical radiographic findings show diffuse, bilateral, ground glass opacities, although sometimes a normal chest radiograph is seen. However, when compared closely with baseline examinations, decreased lung volumes may be evidence for decreased lung compliance (stiff lungs) and, therefore, an interstitial pneumonitis.

- Cytomegalovirus (CMV) can be detected by bronchoscopy with relatively high frequency in HIV-infected patients; however, CMV-positive cultures from bronchial lavage fluid often do not appear related to the clinical picture. Unlike in patients with solid organ transplant immunosuppression, CMV does not appear to contribute directly to the pulmonary disease found in most patients with HIV infection.

- An association between tuberculosis and HIV infection is becoming increasingly evident. Nearly 30% of some populations with tuberculosis are HIV positive. These patients often present with nonspecific constitutional symptoms that are gradual in onset and last for weeks. Clinical and radiographic findings depend on degree of immune compromise. For example, early in the course of HIV infection when the patient's absolute neutrophil count is > 300, a purified protein derivative (PPD) skin test may be positive, with typical chest radiographic findings of upper lobe infiltrates and cavitary opacities. However, in late HIV infection, when the patient's absolute neutrophil count is < 300, the PPD skin test is generally negative, and the chest radiograph shows lymphadenopathy and diffuse heterogeneous parenchymal opacities. Tuberculosis should be suspected in HIV-infected patients when diffuse interstitial lung disease is seen in conjunction with hilar or mediastinal lymph node enlargement. *P. carinii* pneumonia, and other common opportunistic infections do not usually exhibit lymphadenopathy.

- Nontuberculous mycobacterial pulmonary infections also cause serious life-threatening pulmonary disease in patients with advanced HIV-related immunosuppression.

- Diffuse alveolar damage, without a pathogen being detected by either lung biopsy or bronchoalveolar lavage, is seen in up to 40% of patients with AIDS. This is termed "nonspecific interstitial pneumonitis" and it accounts for one third of all episodes of clinical pneumonitis. The clinical features of symptomatic patients with chronic nonspecific interstitial pneumonitis are similar to those of patients with *P. carinii* pneumonia, although histologic findings show less severe alveolar damage in patients with nonspecific interstitial pneumonitis.

- Cryptococcosis is caused by the encapsulated yeast, *Cryptococcosis neoformans*. In patients with AIDS, most cases disseminate and involve the central nervous. Chest radiographic findings are nonspecific and include a solitary pulmonary nodule that may cavitate, multiple nodules, airspace consolidation, or interstitial appearing pneumonia. Mediastinal adenopathy can be seen as well.

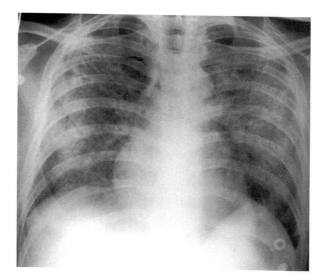

FIGURE 6-19
Anteroposterior chest radiograph of a 39-year-old-man with AIDS shows diffuse bilateral lung opacities typical for *P. carinii* pneumonia.

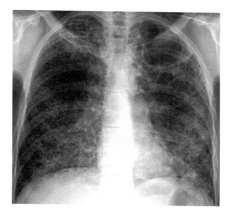

FIGURE 6-20
Posteroanterior chest radiograph of a man with AIDS and a history of chronic and recurrent *P. carinii* pneumonia. Note the coarse interstitial abnormality with lung architectural distortion and large thin-walled cystic spaces, predominately in the upper lobes.

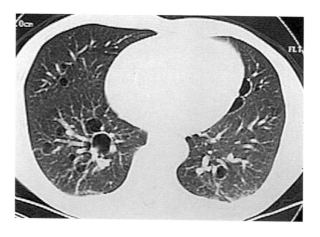

FIGURE 6-21
Chest computed tomography scan through the lower chest of this young man with AIDS shows well-circumscribed, thin walled cysts typical of *P. carinii* pneumonia. In this case, the chest radiograph was normal.

Suggested Reading

Kang EY, Staples CA, McGuinness G, et al. Detection and differential diagnosis of pulmonary infections and tumors in patients with AIDS: value of chest radiography versus CT. *AJR* 1996;166:15–19.

Pneumonia in the Immunocompromised Patient (Non-AIDS)

KEY FACTS

- The pneumonias in the immunocompromised patient tend to be more viral or fungal in etiology and occur in specific patient population subsets such as transplants, immunocompromised, AIDS, diabetics, and so forth (e.g., aspergillosis or CMV in the transplant population).

- Cytomegalovirus is the most common infection (up to 90 %) in solid organ and bone marrow transplant recipients. CMV infection is found between days 30 and 180 in most transplant recipients with diffuse pulmonary infiltrates. In general, opportunistic infections are most common in the period between 1 and 5 months after transplantation. Multiple organism infections almost always involve cytomegalovirus, and they carry a poor prognosis.

- A transient form of nonspecific interstitial pneumonia, radiographically resembling pulmonary edema, may occur during the first 2 weeks after transplantation.

- Heart, heart—lung, and lung transplantation patients offer a slightly different differential diagnosis than other solid organ transplant patients. An abnormal chest radiograph is common during the first month after transplantation; it may be caused by either acute rejection (75%) or, alternatively, lung infection, most commonly CMV pneumonitis. Other causative organisms included *Aspergillus fumigatus*, herpes simplex, *P. carinii*, and *S. aureus*.

- The appearance of CMV infection on radiographs is a generalized, hazy infiltrate, often limited to one lobe. *P. carinii* pneumonia, often combined with CMV infection, usually appears diffusely hazy. Aspergillus infection appears either shaggy and nodular or bibasilar and hazy.

- The CT "halo" sign refers to the finding of ground glass opacity forming a halo around a dense focal area of consolidation. For example, in patients with acute leukemia, the CT halo sign suggests the diagnosis of early invasive pulmonary aspergillosis. This sign is otherwise nonspecific, also being seen with hemorrhagic pulmonary nodules, such as Kaposi's sarcoma metastases or other infections surrounded by a zone of hemorrhagic necrosis.

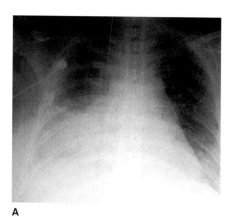

A

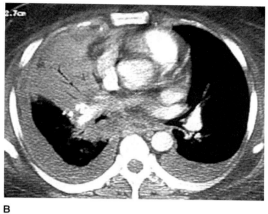

B

FIGURE 6-22   **(A)** Anteroposterior chest radiograph of a 47-year-old woman with severe, poorly controlled diabetes and rapid development of a severe pneumonia with respiratory distress and sepsis shows a nonspecific dense opacification in the right lung base with likely pleural effusion consistent with pneumonia. **(B)** Corresponding CT scan through the lower chest shows bilateral pleural effusions, consolidation of the right middle lobe, and soft-tissue invasion of the right hilar structures and mediastinum by this subsequently proved and eventually fatal fungal infection, in this case mucormycosis.

(continued)

Pneumonia in the Immunocompromised Patient (Non-AIDS) *(Continued)*

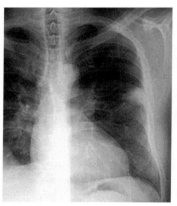

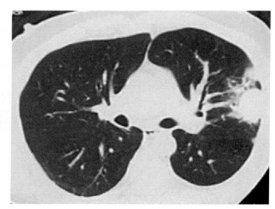

A   B

FIGURE 6-23   Posteroanterior chest radiograph **(A)** and corresponding CT scan **(B)** of a 28-year-old man, who had renal transplantation 3 years before, now presenting with new onset fever and cough productive of black sputum, shows a 3 cm ill-defined, rounded mass in the left upper lobe. Note on the CT scan the halo of ground-glass opacity around the mass. This represents a hemorrhagic necrosis around the area of inflammation, which in this case was caused by mucormycosis.

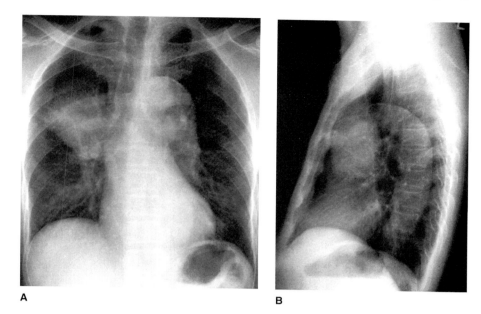

A   B

FIGURE 6-24   Posteroanterior **(A)** and lateral **(B)** chest radiographs of a 64-year-old man shows a wedge-shaped, somewhat masslike opacity in the right upper lobe, which in this case was caused by cryptococcal pneumonia.

Suggested Reading

McAdams HP, Rosado-de-Christianson ML, Templeton PA, et al. Thoracic mycoses from opportunistic fungi: radiologic-pathologic correlation. *Radiographics* 1995;15:271–286.

Bronchiolitis Obliterans-Organizing Pneumonia (BOOP)

KEY FACTS

- Bronchiolitis obliterans-organizing pneumonia (BOOP) is characterized by the presence of granulation tissue within small airways and the presence of areas of organizing pneumonia. It is clinically and pathologically different from obliterative bronchiolitis. BOOP is usually idiopathic. BOOP is, in essence, a noninfectious pneumonia.
- Radiographic features of BOOP almost always are nonspecific, but BOOP tends to be chronic and without response to antibiotic therapy. The CT findings of BOOP are numerous and nonspecific. They include patchy unilateral or bilateral air-space opacification of a ground glass or soft tissue density, small nodular opacities, irregular linear opacities, bronchial wall thickening and dilation, and small pleural effusions. The nodules and air-space consolidation represent different degrees of the same nonspecific inflammatory process that involves the bronchioles, alveolar ducts, and alveoli. CT scans depict the anatomic distribution and extent of bronchiolitis obliterans organizing pneumonia more accurately than do chest radiographs.
- The diagnosis of BOOP is usually made by open lung biopsy.
- BOOP responds to steroid therapy.

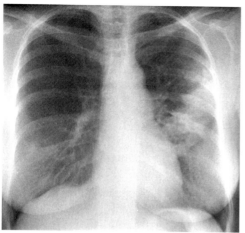

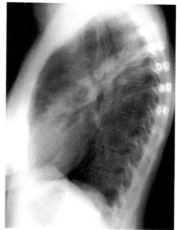

A

B

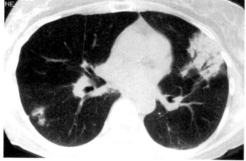

C

FIGURE 6-25

(**A, B**) Posteroanterior (**A**) and lateral (**B**) chest radiograph of a 63-year-old-woman shows a nonspecific area of lung opacification in the left upper lobe. This pneumonia did not respond to antibiotic therapy. (**C**) CT scan through the midchest shows a nonspecific area of consolidation with air-bronchograms in the left upper lobe and a smaller focal area of consolidation in the right lower lobe that was unsuspected on chest radiographs. Open lung biopsy showed this to represent BOOP.

Suggested Reading

Nagai S, Izumi T. Bronchiolitis obliterans with organizing pneumonia. *Current Opinion in Pulmonary Medicine* 1996;2:419–423.

Bronchioloalveolar Carcinoma

KEY FACTS

- Several subtypes of bronchioloalveolar cell carcinoma are based on radiographic appearance: nodular, diffuse, and multifocal.
- The less common (15% to 30%) diffuse form of bronchioloalveolar cell carcinoma carries a worse prognosis than the more common (70% to 85%) focal form.
- Several histologic subtypes of bronchioloalveolar cell carcinoma exist: for example, Clara cell, tall columnar epithelial, and type II pneumocyte.
- Bronchioloalveolar cell carcinomas can produce a large amount of mucus, classically mimicking a pneumonia on chest radiographs. With CT scanning, the lung appears drowned, showing the nonspecific CT angiogram sign, as the lung is essentially drowned in mucus, which can clinically lead to mucorrhea.
- Suspect a bronchioloalveolar cell carcinoma when a chronic pneumonia is present that does not clear as expected or does not have concomitant clinical findings of infection.
- The differential diagnosis for bronchioloalveolar cell carcinoma includes chronic pneumonias (e.g., eosinophilic pneumonia, BOOP), recurrent pneumonias or aspirations, alveolar proteinosis, lymphoma, or pseudolymphoma.
- Bronchioloalveolar carcinoma can also appear as a solitary pulmonary nodule or typical malignant lung mass (see p 108).

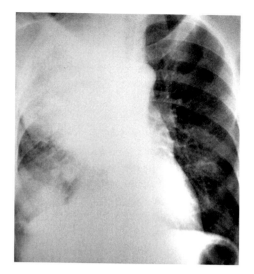

FIGURE 6-26

Anteroposterior chest radiograph of a 70-year-old man with chronic cough productive of excessive mucus shows dense opacification of nearly the whole right lung. This nonspecific appearance was shown to be caused by bronchoalveolar carcinoma.

Suggested Reading

Lee KS, Kim Y, Han J, et al. Bronchoalveolar carcinoma: clinical, histopathologic, and radiologic findings. *Radiographics* 1997;17:1345–1357.

Pulmonary Contusions

KEY FACTS

- The most common traumatic lung injury is a "bruise" or pulmonary contusion.
- Unlike skin bruising, it takes a significant amount of energy absorption to bruise the lung; a pulmonary contusion is a marker of injury severity.
- Pulmonary contusions occur in both blunt and penetrating injuries, with or without rib fractures, and from blast injuries. They are also caused by shearing forces (variable rates of deceleration that compress and stretch the lung).
- Contusions can cause dyspnea, tachycardia, and hypoxia. Hemoptysis is uncommon.
- Mortality rates of up to 31% have been reported in patients with massive pulmonary contusions, and they play a major role in up to 25% of motor vehicle accident fatalities.
- Pulmonary contusions caused by stab or gunshot wounds are usually small and clinically inconsequential, the exception being shotgun wounds that can have a pronounced blast effect.
- Pulmonary contusions are seen radiographically within 6 hours of injury in up to 85% of patients, and in 100% of patients within 12 to 24 hours; they show:
  - Patchy, nonsegmental, ill-defined parenchymal opacity, usually with no anatomic boundary
  - Opacities are peripheral and under the point of injury
  - Opacities can be scattered, or "coup" and "contracoup"
- Pulmonary contusions start clearing in 2 to 3 days—it is a dynamic process that usually resolves within 4 to 5 days (range 1 to 10 days). CT scanning is generally not indicated.
- When new lung parenchymal opacities appear more than 24 hours after injury, strongly consider other causes such as aspiration or superimposed infection.
- A pulmonary contusion can be an independent injury that resolves to leave the chest radiograph normal; however, it can initially mask more serious underlying injuries that only appear as the contusion resolves (e.g., lacerations with resulting pneumatoceles or hematomas).
- Conversely, pulmonary contusions can be masked by other injuries (e.g., pneumothorax, hemothorax).
- Basilar pulmonary contusions, especially with associated rib fractures, should alert the radiologist to associated intra-abdominal injuries.
- A large contusion can result secondary to a blast effect. These types of pulmonary contusions are often more central in locations, unlike those associated with blunt chest wall injuries. Associated injuries include pneumothorax and alveolar rupture with air embolism (leading to early death). Significant lung injury is proportional to the auditory injury and the blast force.

- Lobar contusions occurring after high-velocity (assault or military weapons) gunshot wounds can lead to refractory hypoxemia. Contused lung loses autoregulation and literally shunts blood to itself, away from more normal lung (an intrapulmonary shunt). This type of severe lobar contusion can be treated with lobectomy.

- Shotgun pellets are considered low-velocity projectiles; however, at close range a large blast effect occurs and massive soft-tissue injury can compromise the structural and mechanical integrity of the chest wall.

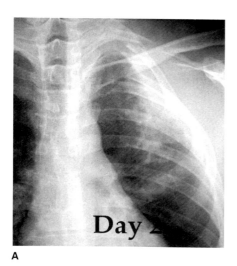 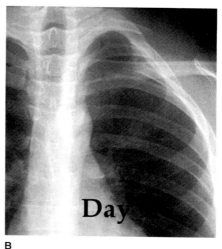

A   **B**

FIGURE 6-27   **(A)** Coned down anteroposterior chest radiograph of a young man involved in a motor vehicle accident shows an ill-defined peripheral opacity in the left upper lobe, directly under several upper rib fractures, typical of a pulmonary contusion. **(B)** A chest radiograph obtained a week later shows the contusion has cleared.

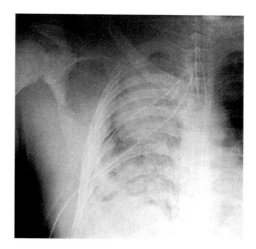

FIGURE 6-28

Anteroposterior chest radiograph of a 43 year-old-man with a rifle wound to the right shoulder. Note the snow storm of metal fragments in the soft tissues. The blast effect from the bullet caused a large right-sided lung parenchymal opacity (contusion).

Suggested Reading

Groskin S. *Radiological, clinical and biomechanical aspects of chest trauma.* Springer Verlag, 1991.

Iatrogenic Causes of Lung Opacification

KEY FACTS

Common iatrogenic causes of lung opacification include malposition of feeding tubes with inadvertent feedings into the lungs, drug toxicity, and radiation pneumonitis. Also, pulmonary infarction can occur after placement of a Swan-Ganz catheter too far into the pulmonary vascular tree.

DRUG TOXICITY

- Drug toxicity is usually a diagnosis of exclusion. A direct temporal relationship with drug exposure and symptoms must be shown.

- The number of drugs known or suspected of causing pulmonary toxicity is steadily increasing and includes bleomycin, procainamide, nitrofurantoin, cyclophosphamide, penicillamine, busulphan, BCNU, amiodarone, mitomycin and methotrexate, among others.

- Toxicity may or may not be dose related. The time course for toxicity of many drugs is variable, from immediate to months or years. Mechanisms of injury are also variable; they include direct pulmonary toxicity and indirect effects through inflammatory or hypersensitivity reactions. Clinical features are similar for most agents—chronic pneumonitis that can lead to lung fibrosis.

RADIATION

- Radiation pneumonitis findings usually are apparent on CT scanning within 16 weeks of radiotherapy, and they are usually detected as early as 4 weeks after completion of radiotherapy.

- Lung injury can progress for several months, but by 6 to 9 months after radiation therapy has been completed, it stabilizes and healing with subsequent scarring ensues.

- Traction bronchiectasis secondary to radiation fibrosis develops from cicatrization and consequent traction reflecting the intense fibrotic nature of late-stage radiation pneumonitis. It is not caused by intrinsic disease of the airways.

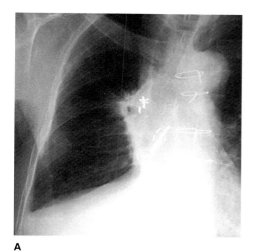

A

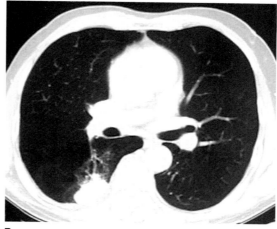

B

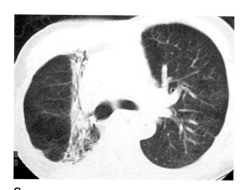

C

FIGURE 6-29

Posteroanterior chest radiograph **(A)** shows evidence of a prior right lower lobectomy. Note the hazy opacity overlying the right hilum and the distortion of the normal anatomic contours. CT scan **(B)** shows the location of the original lung cancer in the right lower lobe. Repeat CT scan 1 year after completion of a course of radiation therapy **(C)** (corresponding with the chest radiograph in **(A)** shows a fibrotic infiltrative process in the medial aspect of the right lung with consequent traction bronchiectasis. Note that the straight, nonanatomic lateral border that marginates the area of fibrosis does not conform to any normal segmental or lobar lung anatomy; rather, it reflects the radiation port, often presenting in a geometric, nonanatomic appearance.

Suggested Reading

Libshitz HF, Shuman LS. Radiation-induced pulmonary change: CT findings. *J Comput Assist Tomogr* 1984;8:15–19.

Asymmetric Pulmonary Edema

KEY FACTS

Asymmetric pulmonary edema is uncommon. It has several radiographic patterns and presentations:

- Focal edema in the right upper lobe. Asymmetric, right upper lobe pulmonary edema is an uncommon phenomenon caused by a mitral regurgitant jet that is preferentially directed into the right upper lobe pulmonary vein, producing focal alteration of the Starling forces and asymmetric accumulation of interstitial fluid. In most of these cases the focal lung opacity can be misdiagnosed as a more common abnormality (e.g., pneumonia). Although it remains difficult to diagnose focal pulmonary edema prospectively using chest radiographs, awareness of its association with mitral regurgitation can alert the clinician to this possibility.

- Relatively diffuse edema is seen with focal sparing of a lobe or multiple segments, such as with pulmonary thromboembolic disease; edema cannot be leaked into lung that is not being perfused.

- Sparing of the upper lobes is usually due to bullous emphysema.

- Apparent unilateral edema may be due to patient positioning; a diffuse edema can shift to one lung as a patient is positioned on that side for prolonged periods.

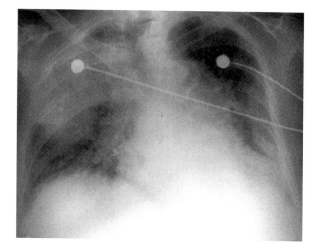

FIGURE 6-30

Anteroposterior chest radiograph of a 78-year-old-woman with mitral regurgitation shows a focal right upper lobe opacity representing focal pulmonary edema.

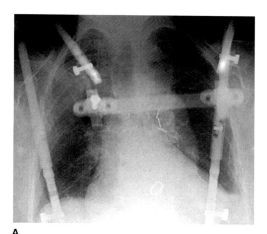

A

FIGURE 6-31

(A) Anteroposterior chest radiograph of an 81-year-old-woman with mitral regurgitation shows development of a hazy new right upper lobe opacity that was originally thought to represent pneumonia, aspiration, or a pulmonary hemorrhage. Compare the right upper lung density with the left. Incidental note of an overlying cervical traction device. **(B)** Chest CT scan showed a focal right upper lobe opacity with distinct enlargement of the right upper lobe pulmonary vessels and thickening of the right upper lobe interlobular septae. Aside from marked left atrial enlargement (not shown), these findings were not present on the preadmission CT done 2 months earlier **(C)**, and they were consistent with focal right upper lobe pulmonary edema secondary to the mitral regurgitation.

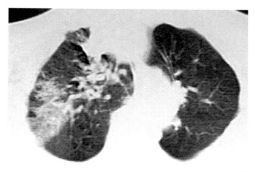

B

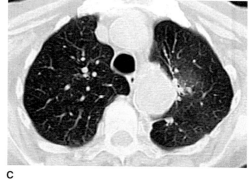

C

Suggested Reading

Gurney JW, Goodman LR. Pulmonary edema localized in the right upper lobe accompanying mitral regurgitation. *Radiology* 1989;171:397–399.

Pulmonary Infarction

KEY FACTS

- Pulmonary infarction is an important vascular cause of lung opacification.
- Infarction associated with pulmonary embolism is rare (< 2%) because of the dual blood supply of the lung (pulmonary arterial and bronchial).
- Lung opacification caused by infarction may consist of hemorrhage and edema, or represent frank tissue necrosis.
- Opacification that can occur typically has a subpleural distribution; it is segmental and most commonly found in the lower lobes. As such, the appearance is nonspecific, frequently interpreted as atelectasis.
- The part of the opacity that abuts the pleura is largest with progressive truncation toward a more central round apex. This appearance is called a "Hampton's hump."
- Wedge-shaped or truncated cone-shaped lesions are useful adjunctive findings of pulmonary embolism in patients who show filling defects on contrast-enhanced spiral CT or angiography.
- The rapidity of resolution of the opacity depends on its cause. Hemorrhagic opacity typically resolves within a week, whereas opacity caused by necrosis requires at least a month.
- Pulmonary infarction is said to melt away like an ice cube, whereas pneumonia resolves in a patchy fashion.

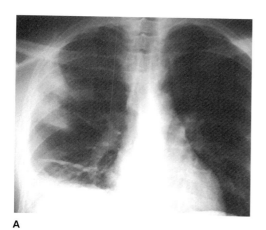

A

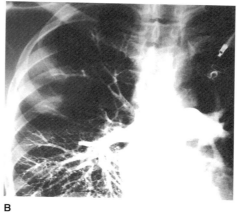

B

FIGURE 6-32 **(A)** Anteroposterior chest radiograph of a 41-year-old-man with recent orthopedic injuries and incapacitation shows a new right upper lobe opacity that was originally thought to represent pneumonia. Workup for pulmonary embolism led to a pulmonary angiogram **(B)** that showed vascular cut-off and almost no blood flow to the areas of lung opacification in the right upper lobe, typical for thromboembolic lung disease, in this case a pulmonary infarction.

Suggested Reading

Greenspan RH, Ravin CE, Polansky SM, et al. Accuracy of the chest radiograph in diagnosis of pulmonary embolism. *Invest Radiol* 1982;17:539–543.

Patterns of Lobar Collapse

- Some common and not so common patterns of lobar collapse.

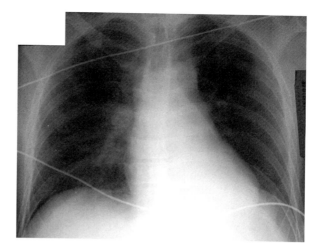

F I G U R E   6 - 3 3

Left lower lobe collapse. Note the dense opacification behind the heart and loss of the left hemidiaphragm contour, the so-called "ivory heart sign."

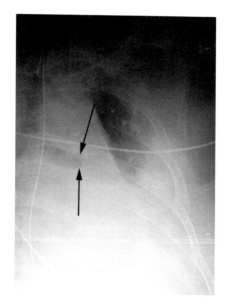

F I G U R E   6 - 3 4

Left lower lobe collapse. In addition to the dense opacification behind the heart and loss of the left hemidiaphragm contour, note the bronchial cut-off sign (*arrows*). The left lower lobe bronchus ends abruptly because of a mucous plug.

(continued)

Patterns of Lobar Collapse (Continued)

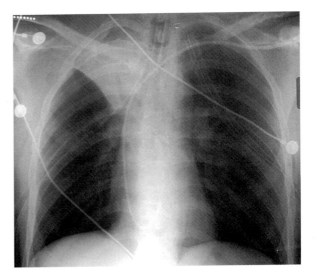

FIGURE 6-35

Right upper lobe collapse. Note the dense opacification and volume loss of the right upper lobe. The minor fissure, representing the bottom of the right upper lobe, is rotated cephalad from the hilum.

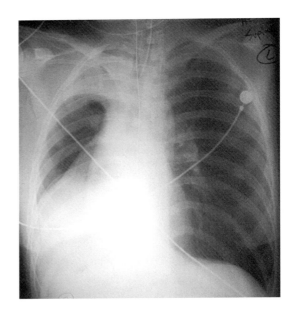

FIGURE 6-36

Right upper and right lower lobe collapse. In this case, it is only the right middle lobe that is aerated.

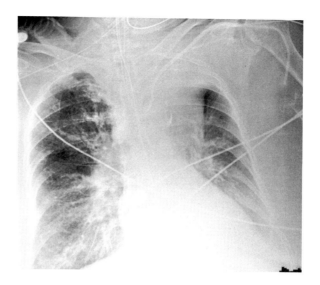

FIGURE 6-37

Partial left upper lobe and left lower lobe. In this case, it is only the lingula (the right middle lobe counterpart) that is aerated. Again, note the ivory heart sign of left lower lobe collapse. The aortic arch is seen only because it is calcified, but otherwise is silhouetted. With a pure left upper lobe collapse, the aortic arch can often been seen with an interface with lung because the left lower lobe hyperinflates behind it, the so-called "luftsichel sign," which is not present in this case because of the left lower lobe collapse.

Suggested Reading

Woodring JH, Reed JC. Radiographic manifestations of lobar atelectasis. *J Thorac Imaging* 1996;11:109–144.

7 Solitary Pulmonary Nodule

Computed Tomography Scanning Technique

KEY FACTS

- There are many ways to "skin a cat" scan. In general, when performing a computed tomography (CT) scan to evaluate a pulmonary nodule, it is usually best to use a standard thick section (e.g., 7 mm) spiral technique to ensure complete coverage of the lung parenchyma. This technique, which is best performed with intravenous (IV) contrast medium, allows detection of other lung nodules and any associated abnormalities such as lymphadenopathy.

- When the slice thickness is about one half or greater than the size of the nodule, an accurate attenuation measurement cannot be obtained because of volume averaging with surrounding lung, within the same pixel. Always obtain several contiguous thin sections (e.g., 1 to 3 mm) through the solitary nodule to get an accurate attenuation reading.

- Some authors have advocated the use of thin sectioning before and after the use of IV contrast to distinguish benign from malignant lesions. This remains controversial and is probably not necessary in all patient populations. This technique would be most helpful in those regions with endemic fungal infections such as histoplasmosis or coccidioidomycosis.

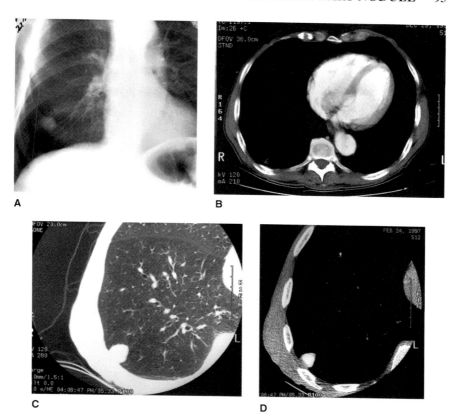

F I G U R E   7 - 1   **(A)** Posteroanterior chest radiograph of a 66-year-old-man with colon cancer shows a 10 mm solitary pulmonary nodule in the right lower lobe. **(B)** A 7 mm spiral computed tomography (CT) scan shows the nodule is noncalcified and, therefore, indeterminate for malignancy. **(C, D)** Thin section (1 mm) CT scan (lung and soft-tissue windows) again shows the nodule; now the dense calcifications of this benign nodule are readily apparent.

Suggested Reading

Swensen SJ. Focal lung disease: CT and high-resolution CT applications. *Radiographics* 1994;14:169–181.

Bronchogenic Cyst

KEY FACTS

- Bronchogenic cysts arise as a duplication of the ventral part of the embryologic foregut.
- Bronchogenic cysts are lined with respiratory epithelium and may contain cartilage.
- Early duplication results in a mediastinal cyst, whereas later duplication causes an intraparenchymal cyst.
- Most series show a strong mediastinal predilection for bronchogenic cysts, but approximately 15% are intraparenchymal.
- Cysts are usually round or ovoid and well-marginated; they can be associated with a bronchus.
- These cysts are typically fluid-filled, but if a connection exists to the tracheobronchial tree because of infection, an air–fluid level can develop.
- Associated findings can include both postobstructive atelectasis or hyperinflation caused by a check-valve mechanism.
- On CT scanning, cysts are homogeneous and do not become enhanced significantly with contrast. Fluid in the cysts is often proteinaceous or hemorrhagic so that CT densities greater than fluid (> 20 HU) are often encountered.
- Small asymptomatic cysts are often treated conservatively. Symptomatic lesions are removed surgically or drained percutaneously.

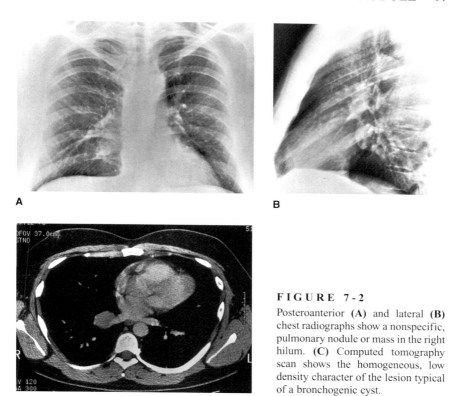

FIGURE 7-2

Posteroanterior **(A)** and lateral **(B)** chest radiographs show a nonspecific, pulmonary nodule or mass in the right hilum. **(C)** Computed tomography scan shows the homogeneous, low density character of the lesion typical of a bronchogenic cyst.

Suggested Reading

Panicek DM, Heitzman ER, Randall PA, et al. The continuum of pulmonary developmental anomalies. *Radiographics* 1987;7:747–772.

Tuberculoma

KEY FACTS

- Tuberculoma is a form of postprimary tuberculosis in which a discrete nodule forms.
- Pathologically, the lesion represents an equilibrium state between the tubercle bacillus and host.
- Tuberculomas are usually well-defined; they may be multiple, and an upper lobe predominance prevails.
- Lesions can grow slowly and reach up to 4 cm in diameter.
- Calcification occurs often; it can be diffuse or confined to the center of the nodule.
- If the nodule cavitates or infiltrate develops in the lung surrounding the nodule, reactivation should be considered.

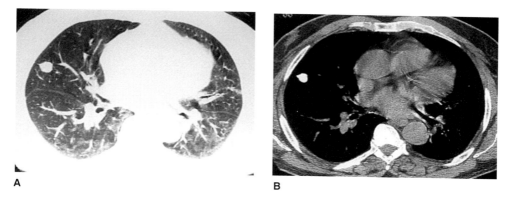

FIGURE 7-3 (**A, B**) Computed tomography scan through the chest (lung and soft-tissue windows) from this older man shows a 12 mm somewhat lobulated but smooth bordered, densely calcified right middle lobe nodule typical of a calcified granuloma, likely from a prior granulomatous infection such as tuberculosis, although histoplasmosis would have a similar appearance.

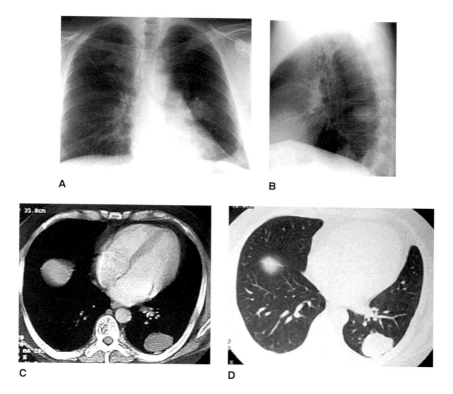

FIGURE 7-4 Posteroanterior (**A**) and lateral (**B**) chest radiograph and corresponding CT scan (**C, D**) (lung and soft-tissue windows from a 41-year-old asymptomatic man, shows a 3 cm mass in the left lower lobe, in this case a proven tuberculoma. Tuberculomas are usually smaller than this example, thus malignancy should always be the initial consideration. This mass was noted to decrease in size with antituberculous therapy.

Suggested Reading

Woodring JH, Vandiviere HM, Fried AM, et al. Update: the radiographic features of pulmonary tuberculosis. *AJR* 1986;146:497–506.

Pulmonary Hamartoma

KEY FACTS

- Pulmonary hamartoma is the most common benign, noninfectious lesion in the lung. Hamartomas are composed of a variety of mesenchymal tissues; cartilage is the most specific. Fat is also common.
- Pulmonary hamartoma usually presents during the fifth decade. Most lesions are less than 4 cm.
- On chest radiography, a lesion may appear as a nonspecific solitary nodule. The presence of popcorn calcification is virtually pathognomonic.
- On CT scanning, attenuation numbers in the fatty range (−80 HU to −120 HU) establish the diagnosis with confidence.
- Carney's triad is the combination of pulmonary hamartoma, leiomyoblastoma, and extra-adrenal paraganglioma.

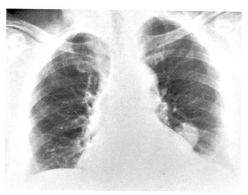

A

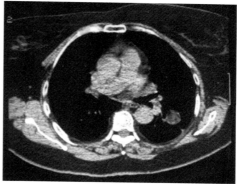

B

FIGURE 7-5   Posteroanterior chest radiograph **(A)** and corresponding CT scan **(B)** of a 51-year-old asyptomatic man, shows a 3 cm mass in the left lower lobe, in this case a proven hamartoma. CT scan shows mixed areas of fat and soft-tissue attenuation typical for a hamartoma.

Suggested Reading

Siegelman SS, Khouri NF, Scott WW, et al. Pulmonary hamartoma: CT findings. *Radiology* 1986;160:313–317.

Bronchial Carcinoid

KEY FACTS

- Bronchial carcinoid is a slow-growing neuroendocrine malignant tumor that is related to small cell lung carcinoma.
- The cell of origin of bronchial carcinoid is believed to be the Kulchitsky cell.
- Bronchial carcinoid rarely causes the carcinoid syndrome.
- Most typical carcinoids are central and occur at bronchial bifurcations. About 20% are found in the peripheral lung.
- Chest radiography can show a central mass that may cause postobstructive atelectasis. A minority of carcinoids present as a solitary pulmonary nodule.
- Carcinoid tumors usually enhance substantially on CT scanning. Large, chunky calcifications occur in 30% of central carcinoids (see images in Chap. 16, p 262).

Suggested Reading

Zweibel BR, Austin JHM, Grimes MM. Bronchial carcinoid tumors: assessment with CT of location and intratumoral calcification in 31 patients. *Radiology* 1991;179:483–486.

Pulmonary Laceration: Pulmonary Hematoma

KEY FACTS

- Pulmonary hematoma results from extensive hemorrhage into a pulmonary laceration. The clot undergoes typical organization and can have a fibrous wall; hence becoming progressively opaque over time.

- Several weeks after an injury, a pulmonary hematoma can begin to appear as (and can be confused with) a solitary pulmonary nodule. However, pulmonary hematomas usually resolve spontaneously and are sometimes called "vanishing lung tumors."

- Pulmonary hematomas can take weeks or months to heal, sometimes with substantial lung scarring.

- Occasionally, pulmonary hematomas form an air crescent sign and can be confused with a mycetoma.

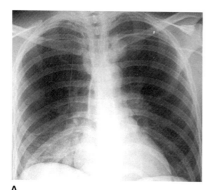 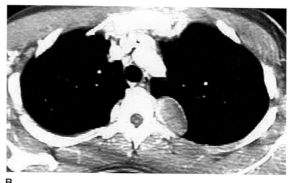

A   **B**

FIGURE 7-6 (A) Anteroposterior chest radiograph of a 24-year-old-man who suffered a motor vehicle accident (MVA) shows a rounded mass in the left upper lobe that apparently developed several days into the hospitalization. Incidental note is made of aspiration in the right lower lobe. (B) CT scan from the same patient shows an ovoid soft-tissue mass in a typical location for a paravertebral, shearing-type, pulmonary laceration or hematoma.

Suggested Reading

Groskin S. Radiological, clinical and biomechanical aspects of chest trauma. Springer Verlag, 1991.

Solitary Pulmonary Nodule Mimics

KEY FACTS

- Pulmonary vessels, seen on end, can be confused with lung nodules.
- A variety of extrapulmonary nodules can appear to be intraparenchymal. Such nodules can be classified as extracorporeal, cutaneous, chest wall-related, or pleural.
- Extracorporeal mimics include overlying monitoring leads or items related to the patient's clothing. Buttons can cause confusion; however, they can often be recognized on the radiograph by their eyeholes.
- The most common cutaneous mimic is a nipple shadow. Often a contralateral nipple shadow is visible. Nipple markers can obviate confusion.
- Other cutaneous lesions such as neurofibromas, nevi, or keloid scars can project over the lungs and appear identical to a solitary lung nodule. A lateral radiograph is often useful to suggest the correct diagnosis. If ambiguity remains, a CT scan is usually definitive.
- Chest wall-related mimics typically are related to the thoracic skeleton. Bone islands or osteochondromas of the rib or scapula, hypertrophy of the first costochondral junction, and callous around healing rib fractures are examples of abnormalities that can be misinterpreted as a solitary pulmonary nodule. Often, a repeat chest radiograph with additional oblique or lordotic projections is confirmatory.
- Breast lesions (e.g., calcified fibroadenomas) can also mimic lung nodules.
- Pleural lesions include fibrous tumor of the pleura and lipoma. They can sometimes be recognized by their tapering margins and their tendency to have one well-defined and one ill-defined border.

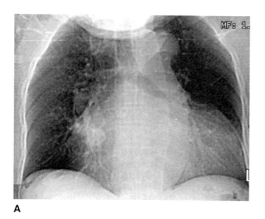
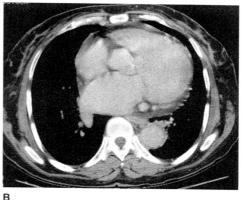

A   B

FIGURE 7-7 **(A)** Computed tomography scout image shows a sharply defined nodule at the right lung base. **(B)** CT scan shows this nodule to represent a dilated pulmonary vein, seen on end, mimicking a lung nodule.

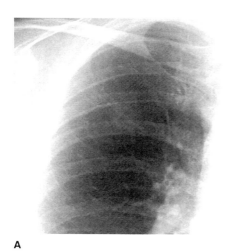
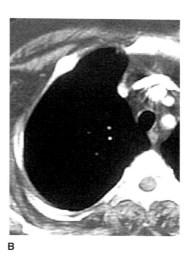

A   B

FIGURE 7-8 **(A)** Posteroanterior chest radiograph, close-up of the right upper lung, shows an ill-defined nodule at the anterior end of the right second rib. **(B)** CT scan shows this nodule to represent callous around a prior 2nd rib fracture.

(continued)

Solitary Pulmonary Nodule Mimics (Continued)

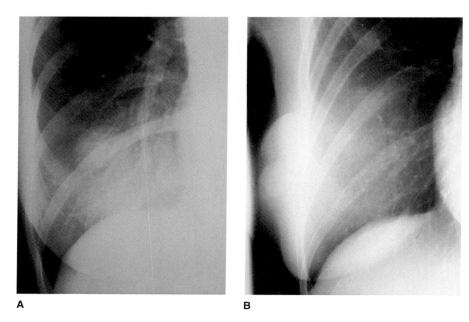

A   B

FIGURE 7-9   **(A)** Posteroanterior chest radiograph, close-up of the right lower lung, shows a nodule with a sharp upper margin. This should suggest an air–tissue interface, perhaps on the skin. **(B)** Right posterior oblique chest radiograph shows this nodule to represent a large breast mass, deforming the normal breast contour.

Suggested Reading
Keats TE. Atlas of normal roentgen variants that may simulate disease, 5th ed. St. Louis: Mosby, 1992.

8 Lung Masses (> 3 cm)

Lung Cancer

KEY FACTS

- Bronchogenic carcinoma is the leading cause of cancer death in the United States (approximately 170,000 in 1993) and is the most common malignancy in the industrialized world.
- Approximately 80% to 90% of cancer deaths are related to cigarette smoking.
- Four histologic types of bronchogenic carcinoma exist: small cell carcinoma (20% to 30%) and the non–small-cell carcinomas; adenocarcinoma (30% to 45%), squamous cell carcinoma (30% to 40%), and large cell carcinoma (10% to 15%).
- Lung cancer presents as a solitary pulmonary nodule in one third of patients. Adenocarcinoma is the most common cell type to produce a solitary pulmonary nodule. These small cancers can be well-marginated, lobulated, or poorly defined. Tumor strands can extend into the surrounding parenchyma, giving rise to a spiculated appearance termed "corona radiata."
- Treatment decisions are partly based on whether the tumor is a small-cell or non–small-cell type.
- Common extrathoracic radiographic manifestions include:
    Metastases to the brain, liver, and adrenal glands
    Paraneoplastic effects such as hypertrophic pulmonary osteoarthropathy
- Calcification within lung cancers on radiographs is distinctly uncommon and is seen in approximately 5% of computed tomography (CT) scans.
- Cavitation occurs most often in squamous cell (20% to 30%) and bronchioloalveolar carcinoma, an adenocarcinoma subtype.
- Computed tomography scanning may show air bronchograms, particularly if the lesion is a bronchioloalveolar carcinoma. CT also evaluates hilar and mediastinal lymph adenopathy, detects metastatic disease (lymphangitic spread, chest wall invasion), and, most importantly, other lung nodules, either as metastases or synchronous lung cancers (1% to 2%).
- The most common location of lung cancer is in the anterior segment of the right upper lobe. The most commonly missed location on chest radiographs is in the right upper lobe. Look extra diligently in this area, especially when a clinical suspicion of malignancy exists.

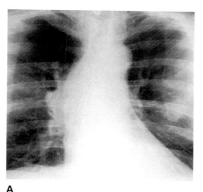
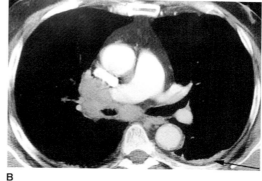

A **B**

FIGURE 8-1   **(A)** Posteroanterior chest radiograph of a 69-year-old man with asbestos exposure and chronic cough shows a right hilar fullness suggestive of a malignancy. **(B)** CT scan confirms the suspicion of lung malignancy, again showing the large right hilar mass. Note the typical noncalcified asbestos-related pleural plaque (*arrow*).

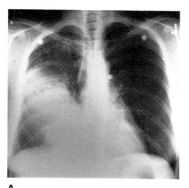
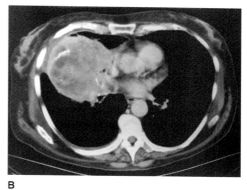

A **B**

FIGURE 8-2   **(A)** Posteroanterior chest radiograph of a 60-year-old woman shows a large cavitating mass in the mid and lower portions of the right lung. This proved to be a large-cell bronchogenic carcinoma. **(B)** CT scan through the mass shows heterogeneous attenuation with both small cavities and unexpected calcification. Calcifications within lung cancers are unusual and likely represent engulfed granulomas or dystrophic calcification.

(continued)

Lung Cancer (Continued)

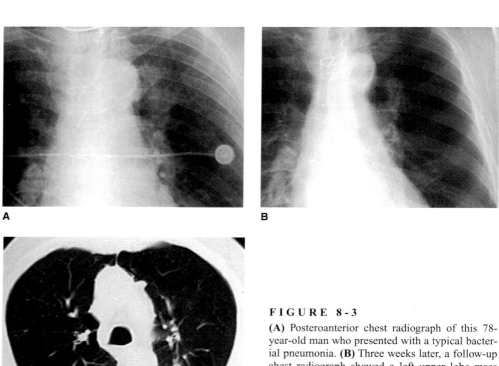

A

B

C

FIGURE 8-3
(A) Posteroanterior chest radiograph of this 78-year-old man who presented with a typical bacterial pneumonia. **(B)** Three weeks later, a follow-up chest radiograph showed a left upper lobe mass that was obscured by the pneumonia. **(C)** Corresponding CT scan showed a spiculated soft-tissue mass in the left upper lobe, abutting the major fissure, which proved to be an adenocarcinoma.

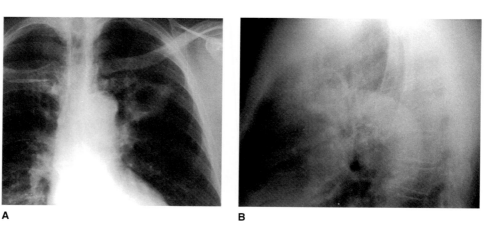

A

B

FIGURE 8-4 Posteroanterior **(A)** and lateral **(B)** chest radiographs of a 70-year-old man with cough and weight loss show a cavitary mass in the left upper lobe, in this case a cavitary squamous cell carcinoma.

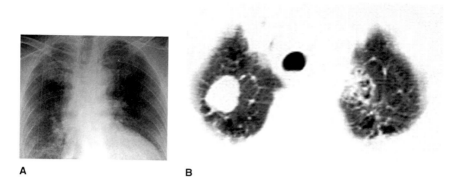

A   B

F I G U R E   8 - 5   **(A)** Posteroanterior chest radiograph of a 60-year-old man who presented for evaluation of chronic cough shows normal senescent changes in the cardiomediastinal contour; no lung masses were noted. **(B)** Corresponding CT scan shows a completely unsuspected large, lobular, somewhat spiculated soft-tissue mass in the right upper lobe that proved to be an adenocarcinoma. Again, the most common location of lung cancer is in the right upper lobe, and the most commonly missed location on chest radiographs is in the right upper lobe.

Suggested Readings

Rosado-de-Christenson ML, Templeton PA, Moran CA. Bronchogenic carcinoma: radiologic-pathologic correlation. *Radiographics* 1994;14:429–446.

White CS, Templeton PA. Radiologic manifestations of bronchogenic cancer. *Clin Chest Med* 1993;4:55–67.

Pancoast Tumor

KEY FACTS

- Pancoast tumors, also called superior sulcus tumors, are primary lung cancers that originate in the lung apex. They typically invade the chest wall or vertebral bodies early in the course of the disease, involving the brachial plexus and causing shoulder and arm pain.
- Pancoast tumors are associated with Horner's syndrome: unilateral miosis, ptosis, and anhydrosis.
- Chest radiographs are of limited value in evaluating chest wall invasion.
- Computed tomography scanning is valuable in detecting bone involvement, but magnetic resonance imaging (MRI) with its multiplanar soft-tissue imaging is best, allowing evaluation and determination of spread of tumor into the spinal cord, nerve roots, brachial plexus, muscle planes, and so forth.
- These tumors differ in location from neurogenic tumors of the posterior mediastinum and are usually distinguishable; they do not arise from the neural foramina (see Chap. 22).

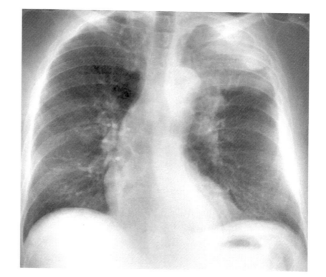

FIGURE 8-6

Posteroanterior chest radiograph of a 76-year-old-man shows a large left apical lung mass typical of a Pancoast (superior sulcus) tumor. No obvious chest wall destruction is seen in this case.

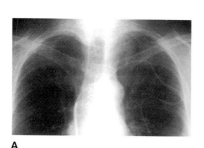

A

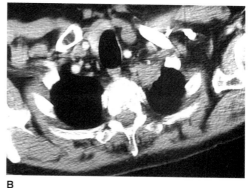

B

FIGURE 8-7 **(A)** Posteroanterior chest radiograph of a 73-year-old man with insidious onset of left shoulder pain who presented with a left-sided Horner's syndrome. Note the vague opacity at the left lung apex. **(B)** CT scan through the apex of the lungs shows a soft-tissue mass in the anterior superior sulcus of the left hemithorax with likely chest wall invasion, typical of a Pancoast-type lung cancer (courtesy of W. Caras, Madigan Army Medical Center).

Suggested Reading

Heelan RT, Demas BE, Caravelli JF, et al. Superior sulcus tumors: CT and MR imaging. *Radiology* 1989;170:637–641.

Rounded Atelectasis

KEY FACTS

- Rounded atelectasis is not a true lung disease, but a result of pleural disease.
- Rounded atelectasis occurs in individuals who have extensive pleural scarring. The focal scarring pulls, retracts, and twists the visceral pleural and adjacent lung into a rounded or lentiform (lens-shaped) mass. Therefore, a thick pleural scar is always seen adjacent to the mass.
- The "mass" has a characteristic CT appearance with a sweeping of bronchovascular structures converging toward the mass, often called a "comet-tail" appearance. Air bronchograms can be seen within the atelectatic parenchyma. Chest radiographic characterization is more difficult, often showing a nonspecific lung mass.
- Any pleural disease that leads to pleural scarring can lead to rounded atelectasis. By far, the most common etiology of rounded atelectasis is asbestos-related pleural disease, although it can occur after any insult that causes pleural scarring, including infections, surgery, or trauma.
- Rounded atelectasis can occur anywhere in the pleural space, and can be multiple.
- Rounded atelectasis can and does increase in size over time, with progressive amounts of scarring and retraction of lung, which can easily be mistaken for a neoplasm. CT scanning should show the characteristic features that allow a "do-not-touch" approach.
- Rounded atelectasis is most often is seen in the lower thorax.

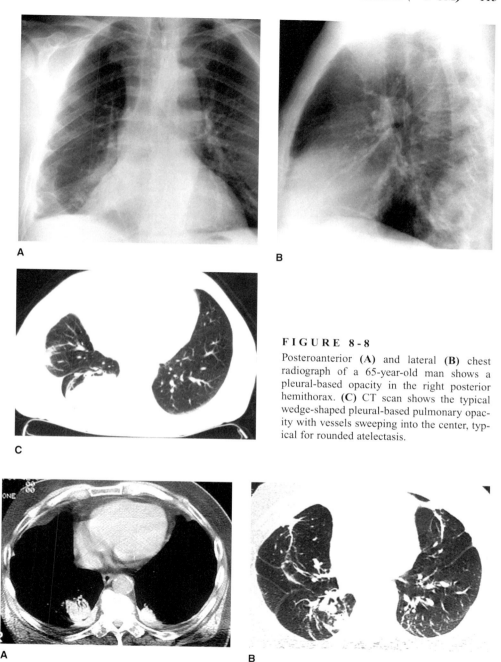

FIGURE 8-8
Posteroanterior (**A**) and lateral (**B**) chest radiograph of a 65-year-old man shows a pleural-based opacity in the right posterior hemithorax. (**C**) CT scan shows the typical wedge-shaped pleural-based pulmonary opacity with vessels sweeping into the center, typical for rounded atelectasis.

FIGURE 8-9 High resolution CT scans. (**A**) Soft-tissue window and (**B**) lung window of this patient with occupational exposure to asbestos show four separate and distinct areas of rounded atelectasis, at slightly different levels, two anteriorly, and the two larger areas, posteriorly. Rounded atelectasis is usually a solitary finding, although it can be multiple, as in this case, and can involve any lobe of the lung, although the most common sites are the inferior or posterior lung bases.

Suggested Reading

Kuhlman JE, Singha NK. Complex disease of the pleural space: radiographic and CT evaluation. *Radiographics* 1997;17:63–79.

Round Pneumonia

- Round pneumonia is an incomplete form of lobar pneumonia that is most common in children. It is thought to occur secondary to the immaturity of collateral ventilation through the pores of Kohn and canals of Lambert.
- In adults, round pneumonia is usually a serendipitous finding that quickly will change to a more typical lobar pneumonia pattern in a matter of hours.
- Round pneumonia can be considered a focal area of infection that spreads outward in a spherical fashion until lobar confines are reached.
- The most common causative organism in children is *Streptococcus* pneumoniae. As with typical lobar pneumonia, air bronchograms may be present.
- In adults, round pneumonia is most likely caused by the common bacterial infections, but it can be caused by fungal organisms such as *Histoplasma*, *Cryptococcus*, *Aspergillus*, and bacteria such as *Nocardia* and *Legionella*.

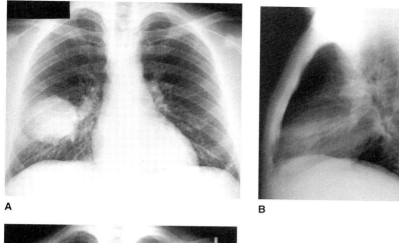

A

B

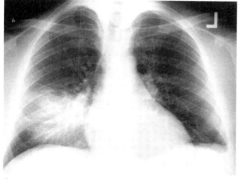

C

FIGURE 8-10
Posteroanterior **(A)** and lateral **(B)** chest radiograph of a 32-year-old man with acute symptoms of pneumonia shows a large round opacity in the right lower lobe. **(C)** PA chest radiograph obtained the next day shows the mass has changed into a more typical appearing lobar pneumonia (see Chap. 6).

Suggested Reading
Rose RW, Ward BH. Spherical pneumonias in children simulating pulmonary and mediastinal masses. *Radiology* 1973;106:179.

9 Multiple Pulmonary Nodules

Pulmonary Metastases

KEY FACTS

- Most common primary sites of malignancy to metastasize to the lung are breast, kidney, colon, prostate, head and neck, and the lung itself.
- The nodules are often subpleural and basilar in location because of the greater blood flow (up to three times more than apices).
- The histology of cavitary metastases is most frequently squamous cell carcinoma. The most common primary tumor sites are the cervix and the head and neck. Colon carcinoma is the most common primary tumor to cause cavitary metastatic adenocarcinoma in the lungs.
- Calcification or ossification of metastases is usually caused by primary osteosarcoma or chondrosarcoma.
- Ill-defined metastases can occur with vascular primary neoplasms such as choriocarcinoma and adenocarcinoma.
- Computed tomography (CT) scanning, especially spiral (helical) CT scanning, typically shows many more nodules than the chest radiograph. CT scanning also shows calcification or cavitation to better advantage.
- On CT, a vessel can be found leading directly into the metastatic nodule. This finding, termed the "feeding vessel" sign, is suggestive of the hematogenous origin of the metastasis.

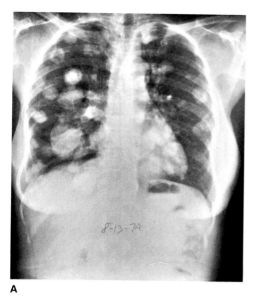

A

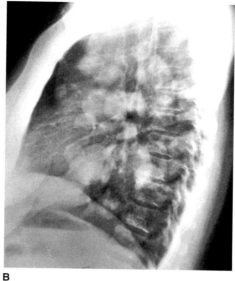

B

FIGURE 9-1   Posteroanterior (A) and lateral (B) chest radiographs demonstrate multiple well-defined lung nodules. Biopsy revealed metastases from adenocarcinoma of the parotid.

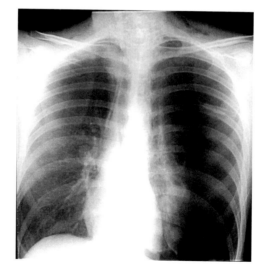

FIGURE 9-2

Posteroanterior chest radiograph of a 21-year-old man with a history of osteosarcoma of the lower extremity, who presented with sudden shortness of breath. A large left pneumothorax is seen. Closer inspection shows several sharply defined nodules in the collapsed left lung, typical of metastatic disease. Osteosarcoma metastases to the lung can cause a spontaneous pneumothorax.

Suggested Reading

Davis SD. CT evaluation for pulmonary metastases in patients with extrathoracic malignancy. *Radiology* 1991;180:1–12.

Invasive Pulmonary Aspergillosis

KEY FACTS

- Aspergillosis has three different clinical presentations: saprophytic, allergic, and invasive, occurring along a spectrum of host immune response, from hyperimmune (allergic, Chap. 16) to normal (saprophytic, Chap. 12) to hypoimmune (invasive).

- The saprophytic form consists of a collection of mycelia that develops in a preexisting cavity. The lesion is often called a mycetoma or "fungus ball." The host immune system is usually normal.

- The allergic form, also known as allergic bronchopulmonary aspergillosis (ABPA), is caused by a hypersensitivity reaction and typically is associated with asthma and eosinophilia. It manifests radiographically as central bronchiectasis and mucus plugging (finger-in-glove).

- The invasive form occurs in patients who have severe immunocompromise; it is characterized by vascular invasion. Patients affected include those with hematologic disorders, particularly leukemia and lymphoma; transplant patients; and, less commonly, those with acquired immune deficiency syndrome (AIDS).

- The most frequent radiographic manifestation of invasive pulmonary aspergillosis is of nonspecific single or multiple pulmonary nodules or opacifications. A miliary or diffuse small nodular pattern is less common.

- Pulmonary nodules develop in previously normal lung parenchyma and enlarge slowly. Neutropenia appears to be a substantial factor in fostering growth of the nodules. In patients who recover from the neutropenia (e.g., leukemics), the nodule frequently cavitates along its outer margin, a relatively nonspecific phenomenon termed "the air-crescent sign."

- Computed tomography (CT) scanning may show nodules that are not evident on the chest radiograph. CT can also show a halo of ground glass attenuation around a nodule, a relatively nonspecific finding, which in the proper clinical setting represents hemorrhagic necrosis, often a precursor to frank cavitation.

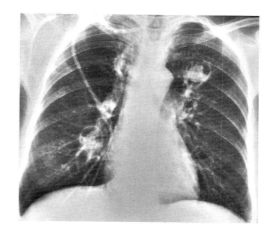

FIGURE 9-3

Posteroanterior chest radiograph shows three cavitary pulmonary nodules in a patient with leukemia and invasive pulmonary aspergillosis. Note the air-crescent configuration of the cavitation.

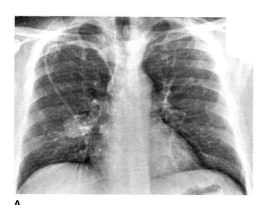

A

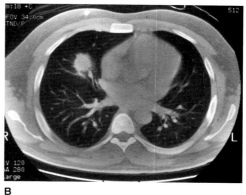

B

FIGURE 9-4   **(A)** Posteroanterior chest radiograph of a 29-year-old man with leukemia and invasive pulmonary aspergillosis shows a rounded mass overlying the right hilum. A double lumen central venous catheter is in the expected position. **(B)** Corresponding CT scan through the right middle lobe shows the mass has a halo of increased ground glass attenuation representing hemorrhagic necrosis, a clue to the diagnosis of invasive aspergillosis.

Suggested Readings

Aquino SL, Kee ST, Warnock ML, et al. Pulmonary aspergillosis: imaging findings with pathologic correlation. *AJR* 1994;163:811–815.

Greene R. The pulmonary aspergilloses: three distinct entities or a spectrum of disease. *Radiology* 1981;140:527–530.

Multiple Parenchymal Hematomas

KEY FACTS

- Pulmonary hematomas usually develop following major blunt or penetrating chest trauma.
- Mechanism of pulmonary hematoma is parenchymal shearing with pulmonary laceration. A laceration that fills with air is called a "pneumatocele." A "hematoma" is a laceration that fills with blood.
- Pulmonary hematoma may not be visible for several hours or longer because of the surrounding parenchymal opacity.
- Pulmonary hematoma usually requires weeks to months to resolve; it is often the only late evidence of trauma.
- On chest radiographs, a pulmonary hematoma manifests as one or more well-defined nodules or masses. The lesion is usually less than 5 cm in diameter. CT shows the lesion more clearly.
- Lesion can usually be treated conservatively.

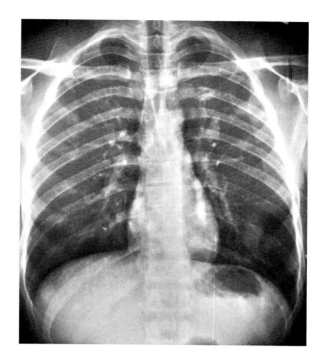

FIGURE 9-5
Posteroanterior chest radiograph shows three ovoid, well-demarcated parenchymal lesions in a patient who suffered blunt chest trauma four weeks earlier. Subsequent radiographs showed a slow resolution of the lesions over a period of 6 months.

Suggested Reading

Williams JR. The vanishing lung tumor—pulmonary hematoma. *AJR* 1959;81:296.

Nodular Pulmonary Amyloidosis

KEY FACTS

- Amyloid is a proteinaceous substance that when stained with Congo Red shows green birefringence in polarized light.

- Primary amyloidosis and multiple myeloma cause a systemic disease. A reactive systemic form is usually caused by rheumatoid arthritis or tuberculosis.

- Systemic amyloidosis can show lung involvement, whereas localized or isolated forms of amylidosis occur in the lung, heart, or kidneys.

- Most patients with systemic disease have normal chest radiographs. Infrequently, radiographs show an increase of interstitial markings.

- Primary pulmonary amyloidosis is a rare disease that occurs in three forms: tracheobronchial, nodular parenchymal, and diffuse parenchymal or alveolar septal.

- The tracheobronchial form typically causes diffuse irregular large airway narrowing and can lead to obstructive atelectasis.

- In the diffuse parenchymal or alveolar septal form, amyloid deposition in the lung is often widespread, involving small blood vessels and the parenchymal interstitium, and multifocal small nodules of amyloid may be present. The diffuse parenchymal or alveolar septal form of amyloidosis is least common, but it is clinically most significant. Patients with diffuse parenchymal amyloidosis are more likely to die of respiratory failure than are patients with the two other forms of the disease.

- Radiologically, the diffuse parenchymal or alveolar septal form of amyloid appears as nonspecific diffuse interstitial or alveolar opacities, which once established change little over time. The abnormal areas can calcify or, rarely, show frank ossification. The diffuse parenchymal abnormality can be predominantly nodular, but diffuse inhomogeneous opacities may also be seen.

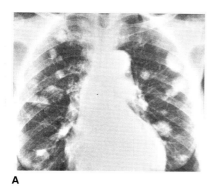
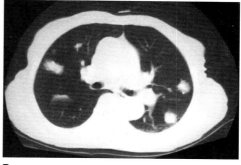

A   **B**

FIGURE 9-6   Posteroanterior **(A)** and lateral **(B)** chest radiographs demonstrate multiple bilateral pulmonary nodules, in this case, due to amyloidosis. On chest CT, it is evident that the nodules are calcified.

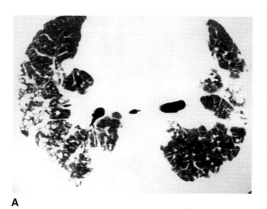
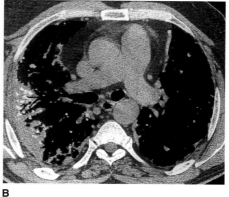

A   **B**

FIGURE 9-7   **(A)** High resolution CT scan (lung window) through the midlung zone from this middle aged man with alveolar septal amyloidosis shows reticular opacities and multiple small nodular opacities scattered through the lungs, but having a peripheral predominance. Confluent subpleural opacities are also noted. Some interlobular septal thickening is seen. **(B)** Soft-tissue window setting shows multiple discrete foci of calcification within the large confluent subpleural opacities.

Suggested Reading

Graham CM, Stern EJ, Finkbeiner WE, et al. HRCT appearance of diffuse alveolar septal amyloidosis. *AJR* 1992;158:265–267.

Multiple Septic Emboli

KEY FACTS

- Multiple septic emboli can occur after hematogenous spread of infected material into the lung.

- The most common sources of septic emboli are tricuspid valve endocarditis in intravenous drug users; infected central venous catheters and surgical hardware; and septic thrombophlebitis.

- The most common organisms are *Staphylococcus aureus*, *Streptococcus viridans*, and *S. pneumoniae*.

- The diagnosis is usually confirmed by culturing organisms from blood or catheter tips.

- Most common chest radiographic manifestation is multiple pleural-based, round, or wedge-shaped parenchymal opacities that have a basilar predilection because of the greater blood flow in the lung bases.

- On chest radiographs, lesions are often in varying states of cavitation, depending on their chronicity. With CT scanning, up to 50% of lesions show cavitation. The appearance can be similar to that of Wegener's granulomatosis. The clinical presentation is useful in distinguishing the two processes.

- Computed tomography scans can show a vessel leading into the parenchymal opacity (feeding vessel sign), which suggests a hematogenous origin of the process.

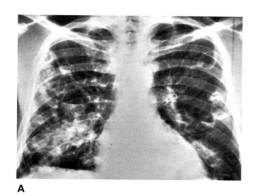

A

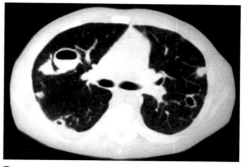

B

FIGURE 9-8   (A) Posteroanterior chest radiograph shows bilateral peripheral pulmonary nodules, many of which are cavitary. (B) CT scan shows the lesion more clearly. Note the different sizes and degrees of cavitation.

Suggested Reading

Kuhlman JE, Fishman EK, Teigen C. Pulmonary septic emboli: diagnosis with CT. *Radiology* 1990;174:211–213.

Nodular Sarcoidosis

KEY FACTS

- Sarcoidosis is a systemic disease that causes formation of noncaseating granulomas in multiple organs, including the skin, bone, heart, eyes, meninges, and, especially, the lungs. The cause is unknown.
- Intrathoracic nodal disease is most common. Approximately one third of patients with nodal disease ultimately develop lung parenchymal disease.
- On chest radiographs, reticulonodular opacities occur in approximately 80% of patients with parenchymal disease; they are the most common parenchymal manifestation. A consolidative (alveolar) pattern occurs in about 20% of patients.
- Histopathologic correlate of an alveolar pattern is caused by either compression of alveoli by interstitial sarcoidosis or by direct alveolar filling.
- A chest radiographic nodular pattern of sarcoidosis occurs in 2% of affected patients. These nodules are typically ill-defined and multiple, and they can reach 5 cm or more in diameter.
- With CT scanning, air bronchograms can be identified within the nodules. Frank cavitation (necrosis) of nodules is rare.
- As with most cases of sarcoidosis, nodular sarcoidosis has a variable prognosis. The nodules can persist or regress.

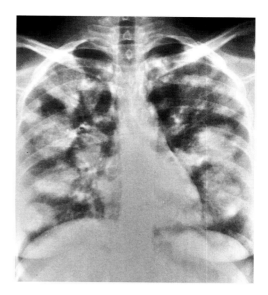

FIGURE 9-9
Posteroanterior chest radiograph of a patient with sarcoidosis shows multiple ill-defined nodules that measure approximately 5 cm in diameter.

Suggested Readings

Freundlich IM, Libshitz HI, Glassman LM, et al. Sarcoidosis: typical and atypical thoracic manifestations and complications. *Clin Radiol* 1970;21:376–383.

Rockoff SD, Rohatgi PK. Unusual manifestations of thoracic sarcoidosis. *AJR* 1985;144: 513–528.

Wegener's Granulomatosis

KEY FACTS

- Wegener's granulomatosis (WG) is characterized by a necrotizing granulomatous vasculitis of both upper and lower airways, diffuse small vessel vasculitis, and focal glomerulonephritis.
- The cause of WG is unknown, but it may reflect an autoimmune disorder.
- If only the lungs are involved, the disease is termed "limited" WG.
- Mean age at presentation is in the fifth decade with a slight male predilection.
- Most patients have a positive cytoplasmic antineutrophilic cytoplasmic antibody (cANCA) test.
- Chest radiographs typically show one to several ill-defined nodular masses that measure 2 to 4 cm in diameter and cavitate in up to 50% of patients. The nodular masses appear to be in different stages of evolution: younger, smaller opacities and larger, older cavitating regions (especially with serial examinations).
- Some patients present with focal or widespread lung opacification.
- Additional manifestations of WG include diffuse pulmonary hemorrhage, tracheal narrowing (see also Chap. 16), subglottic stenosis, and pleural effusions.

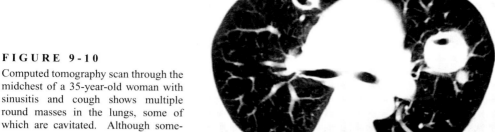

FIGURE 9-10
Computed tomography scan through the midchest of a 35-year-old woman with sinusitis and cough shows multiple round masses in the lungs, some of which are cavitated. Although somewhat nonspecific, these masses are typical of Wegener's granulomatosis.

Suggested Reading

Farrelly CA. Wegeners granulomatosis: a radiological review of the pulmonary manifestations at initial presentation and during relapse. *Clin Radiol* 1982;33:545–551.

Rheumatoid Nodules

KEY FACTS

- Rheumatoid nodules in the lungs are necrobiotic nodules that are a manifestation of rheumatoid arthritis. A male predominance is seen.
- Pathologically, the nodule is identical to that found in the subcutaneous tissues.
- Lung nodules typically occur in patients with advanced rheumatoid arthritis.
- Rheumatoid lung nodules are usually asymptomatic, but they occasionally rupture into the pleural cavity and can cause pneumothorax.
- On chest radiographs, rheumatoid nodules usually appear as one to several nodules, often with a subpleural predilection.
- The combination of rheumatoid nodules and coal worker's pneumoconiosis is termed "Caplan's syndrome."

Suggested Reading

Anaya JM, Diethelm L, Ortiz LA, et al. Pulmonary involvement in rheumatoid arthritis. *Semin Arthritis Rheum* 1995;24:242–254.

Kaposi's Sarcoma

KEY FACTS

- Prior to the advent of AIDS, Kaposi's sarcoma was an uncommon and indolent neoplasm that affected older men of Jewish or Mediterranean origin.
- AIDS-associated Kaposi's sarcoma is very aggressive and is often the initial manifestation of AIDS.
- Kaposi's sarcoma in patients with AIDS occurs in both the homosexual and heterosexual population. The causative agent is thought to be a sexually transmitted virus.
- Kaposi's sarcoma predominantly affects the skin; however, the lungs, gastrointestinal tract, and lymph nodes are other sites of involvement.
- Nearly all patients who have Kaposi's sarcoma of the lung also have skin involvement.
- On chest radiographs, opacities caused by Kaposi's sarcoma tend to be coarser and less uniform than those caused by *Pneumocystis carinii* pneumonia. The opacities, which often radiate from the hilum, may coalesce and form poorly marginated nodules.
- Pleural effusions are often present. Lymph node enlargement can occur, but typically it is not massive.
- Computed tomography scans more clearly show the perihilar and peribronchovascular distribution of pulmonary Kaposi's sarcoma.

(continued)

Kaposi's Sarcoma (Continued)

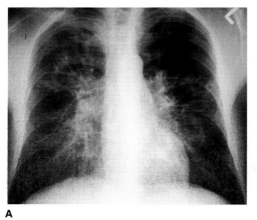

A

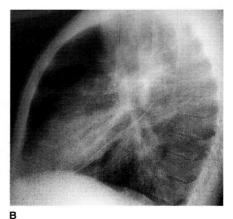

B

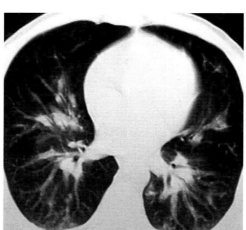

C

FIGURE 9-11
Posteroanterior **(A)** and lateral **(B)** chest radiographs of a 42-year-old man with AIDS and Kaposi's sarcoma shows ill-defined opacities radiating from both hila. **(C)** CT scan shows the tumor growing along the bronchovascular bundles, which appear larger than expected. Also seen are poorly marginated nodules along the bronchovascular bundles.

Suggested Reading

Sivit CJ, Schwartz AM, Rockoff SD. Kaposi's sarcoma of the lungs in AIDS: radiologic-pathologic analysis. *AJR* 1987;148:25–28.

Multiple Pulmonary Arteriovenous Malformations

KEY FACTS

- Pulmonary arteriovenous malformations (AVM) are caused by direct communication of a pulmonary artery and pulmonary vein.

- Approximately 50% of patients with pulmonary AVM have Osler-Weber-Rendu (OWR) syndrome; 25% of patients with OWR have one or more pulmonary AVMs.

- Osler-Weber-Rendu syndrome is transmitted by an autosomal dominant gene.

- Other manifestations of OWR, also termed "hereditary hemorrhagic telangiectasia," include telangiectasias of the skin and mucous membranes.

- Although the AVMs are presumed to be present at birth, they usually do not manifest until adulthood.

- Patients with OWR may present with symptoms identical to those with solitary pulmonary AVM, including lung parenchymal bleeding or brain lesion. They may also develop bleeding from gastrointestinal tract telangiectasias.

- The imaging findings in OWR are similar to those for solitary pulmonary AVM except that multiple lesions are often found.

- Embolotherapy is effective for one or a few lesions. Surgery may be necessary if multiple lesions are limited to one part of the lung.

(continued)

Multiple Pulmonary Arteriovenous Malformations
(Continued)

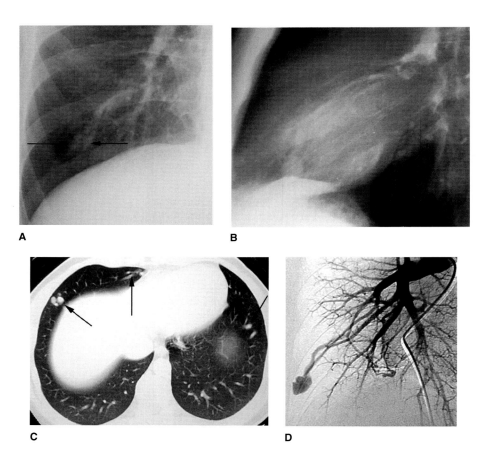

FIGURE 9-12   (A) Close-up radiograph of the right lower lung of a 26-year-old man who presented with a brain abscess shows an ill-defined nodule in the right middle lobe (*arrows*). (B) The lateral view suggests the possibility of feeding vessels and draining veins. (C) CT scan through the lung bases shows this mass to represent an arteriovenous malformation. Incidentally, three other AVMs were also found (*arrows*). These were confirmed by pulmonary angiography (D) and subsequently embolized.

Suggested Reading

Hodgson CH, Burchell HB, Good CA, et al. Hereditary hemorrhagic telangectasia and pulmonary arteriovenous fistula. *N Engl J Med* 1958;261:625–636.

10   Miliary Pattern

Histoplasmosis

KEY FACTS

- Histoplasmosis is an infection secondary to the fungus *Histoplasma capsulatum*.
- Endemic areas of infection include the Mississippi and Ohio river valleys, which cover up to one third of the area of the continental United States, making histoplasmosis very common.
- Histoplamosis is usually a subclinical infection that occurs after inhaling the organism. One to several lung parenchymal granulomas form and are associated with hilar or mediastinal lymph node involvement. All lesions usually calcify.
- The lung granulomas, which vary in size from pinpoint to several centimeters in diameter, are usually an incidental chest radiographic finding.
- With computed tomography (CT) scanning, calcified granulomas are frequently seen within the liver, spleen, or both.

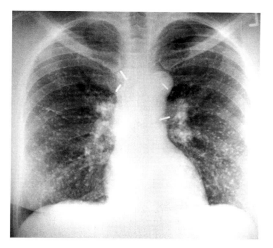
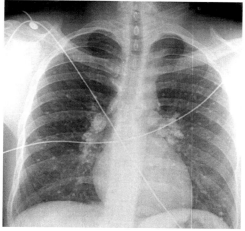

FIGURES 10-1 and 10-2   Anteroposterior chest radiographs from two different patients with miliary histoplasmosis show innumerable small, dense nodules throughout the lungs. Both cases show calcified hilar lymph nodes as well.

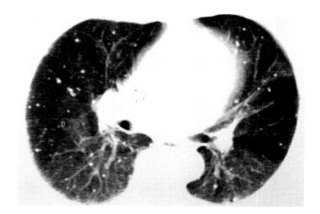

FIGURE 10-3

Computed tomography scan through the lower chest of this 72-year-old man shows many small, densely calcified lung nodules typical of a healed more extensive spread of histoplasmosis.

Suggested Reading

Boyars MC, Zwischenberger JB, Cox CS Jr. Clinical manifestation of pulmonary fungal infections. *J Thorac Imaging* 1991;7:12–22.

Varicella

KEY FACTS

- Varicella-zoster virus can cause either chickenpox or shingles. Varicella pneumonia is an acute chickenpox pneumonia that usually occurs in adults who have severe cutaneous disease. Varicella pneumonia is uncommon in children; 90% of affected patients are aged 19 years or older. Only rarely does an older patient with herpes zoster present with varicella pneumonia.

- Varicella pneumonia is more prevalent in immunocompromised patients, particularly those with hematologic malignancies. Pregnant patients are also vulnerable to varicella pneumonia.

- Clinical and radiographic features of varicella pneumonia develop 2 to 5 days after the skin lesions. The chest radiograph most commonly shows a diffuse nodular infiltrate with a peribronchovascular distribution, probably reflecting contiguous spread from tracheobronchitis. The nodules are ill-defined, usually less than 5 mm in diameter, and may form a miliary pattern. Pleural effusion and hilar adenopathy can be present.

- The radiographic appearance can be similar to other interstitial processes such as sarcoidosis, miliary tuberculosis, or lymphangitic carcinomatosis, but varicella pneumonia is usually not a diagnostic dilemma in light of the clinical presentation. Chest radiographic clearing can take from 10 days to several months, or even years, with residual widespread fibrotic nodules. A sequela of varicella pneumonia is widespread multiple tiny calcified nodules measuring 2 to 3 mm; less than 2% of patients with varicella pneumonia develop these calcifications.

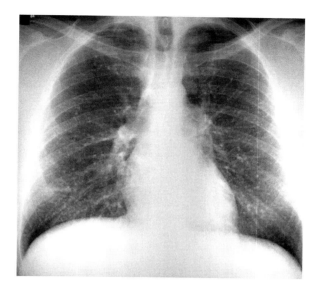

FIGURE 10-4
Anteroposterior chest radiograph of a 35-year-old-man shows innumerable small, dense nodules throughout the lungs as residua of varicella pneumonia.

Suggested Reading

Sargent EN, Carson MJ, Reilly ED. Roentgenographic manifestations of varicella pneumonia with postmortem correlation. *AJR* 1966;98:305–317.

Miliary Tuberculosis

KEY FACTS

- Less than 5% of patients with primary tuberculosis do not contain the primary site of infection; the mycobacterial infection spreads hematogenously. These patients usually have an impaired immune system. This form of tuberculosis is called miliary tuberculosis.

- Most patients with miliary tuberculosis go on to heal, but during the acute infection, chest radiographs show innumerable ill-defined nodular opacities about 3 to 5 mm in diameter. The miliary nodules are not calcified.

- After the acute infection heals, the radiograph may return to normal, or scattered residua of the small ill-defined nodules may exist; they are not evidently calcified.

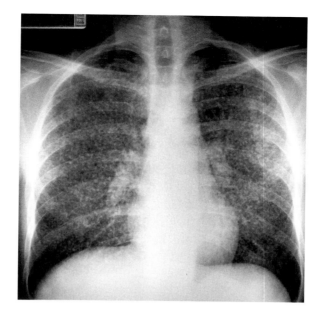

FIGURE 10-5
Anteroposterior chest radiograph of a 47-year-old-man with subacute miliary tuberculosis shows innumerable small, dense nodules throughout the lungs.

Suggested Reading

Buckner CB, Walker CW. Radiologic manifestations of adult tuberculosis. *J Thorac Imaging* 1990;5:28–37.

Silicosis

KEY FACTS

- Silicosis is caused by inhalation of free silica.

- Occupational exposure occurs in miners, quarry workers, foundry workers, sandblasters, and workers in the ceramics industry. At least 10 years of exposure is usually required before radiographic abnormalities become evident.

- The pathologic lesion is the silicotic nodule, which contains silica particles surrounded by dense concentric collagenous material.

- The chest radiographic appearance of simple silicosis is that of multiple lung nodules that range in size from 1 to 10 mL.

- The nodules have a predilection for the upper lobes, particularly the posterior segments. Nodules can calcify. On high-resolution CT, nodules may be located centrilobularly and subpleurally.

- Lymphadenopathy can be present: lymph nodes can calcify diffusely or in a rimlike pattern, the so-called "eggshell calcification" (also seen in sarcoidosis and treated lymphoma).

- If the nodules coalesce to a masslike density that exceeds 1 cm, the term "progressive massive fibrosis" (PMF) is used. PMF defines complicated silicosis.

- Progressive massive fibrosis tends to start peripherally and extend toward the hila as additional nodules are incorporated. Radiographically, PMF appears as an irregular mass or masses, often bilateral, in the mid or upper lung zones that may calcify or cavitate. Paracicatricial emphysema is usually seen around the fibrotic masses.

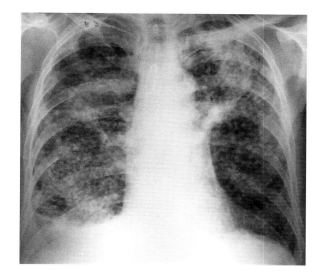

FIGURE 10-6
Posteroanterior chest radiograph of a 64-year-old-man who worked as a quartz miner for 30 years shows innumerable small, dense nodules throughout the lungs and formation of progressive massive fibrosis in the upper lobes.

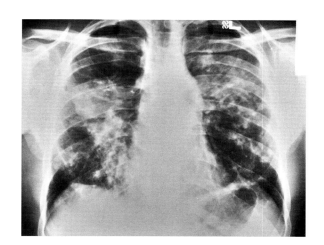

FIGURE 10-7
Posteroanterior chest radiograph shows multiple nodules and masses from a patient with long-standing complicated silicosis (progressive massive fibrosis).

Suggested Reading

Gamsu G. CT and HRCT of pneumoconiosis. *J Occup Med* 1991;33:794–796.

11 Interstitial Lung Diseases

Usual Interstitial Pneumonia (Fibrosing Alveolitis)

KEY FACTS

- Usual interstitial pneumonia (UIP) is a pathologic term. Its cause varies, ranging from collagen vascular disease, to asbestos exposure, to unknown agents. Most evidence suggests that it arises from a derangement of the immune system. In those patients with pathologic features of UIP from unknown cause, the term "idiopathic pulmonary fibrosis" (IPF) is applied.

- Desquamative interstitial pneumonia is considered by some experts to be an earlier, more favorable, stage in the continuum of parenchymal changes that ultimately lead to fibrosis (UIP). However, this is controversial.

- Usual interstitial pneumonia occurs most frequently in middle-aged patients with an approximate equal gender predilection. Diagnosis is suggested by computed tomography (CT) or high resolution CT (HRCT), especially the later stages. Tissue sampling, by thoracoscopy or open lung biopsy, is often needed to diagnose earlier stages of disease. Long-term prognosis is poor.

- Radiographically, early UIP is not detected. As the disease progresses, radiographs show mild reticular changes, often at the lung bases. More advanced disease show coarse, more diffuse reticulonodular abnormalities, accompanied by low lung volumes.

- Computed tomography, especially HRCT, shows changes of UIP much earlier than radiographs and correlates better with clinical symptoms.

- Features of early lung fibrosis seen on HRCT include thickening of the interlobular septa, ill-defined centrilobular nodular opacities, a fine intralobular reticular pattern, ground glass opacity, parenchymal bands, subpleural line, and lobular architectural distortion. The changes can be diffuse but have a basilar and peripheral predominance. In early disease, prone CT scanning may be necessary to distinguish these fibrotic changes from those of normal, gravity-related dependent density.

- Late stage UIP shows multiple confluent lung cysts that have a "honeycomb" appearance.

- In patients with end-stage UIP, honeycombing occurs in association with increased distortion of lung architecture and traction bronchiectasis.

Scleroderma Lung

KEY FACTS

- Specific sites of disease associated with multisystemic collagen vascular disease scleroderma (progressive systemic sclerosis) include skin changes, Raynaud's phenomenon, esophageal dysmotility, and lung fibrosis.
- The female-to-male distribution is approximately 3:1.
- Pathologically, typical features of UIP are seen. Because a cause exists (a collagen vascular disease), the term "idiopathic pulmonary fibrosis" is not applied, although the appearance is both pathologically and radiologically indistinguishable from other causes of UIP.
- As with other lung fibroses, the chest radiograph shows low lung volumes and basilar reticular or reticulonodular interstitial opacities. Severe cases show large cystic spaces (honeycombing).
- Other radiographic findings include enlargement of the pulmonary arteries caused by pulmonary arterial hypertension, aspiration pneumonia, and esophageal dilation.
- Findings on HRCT are as with any of the causes of usual interstitial pneumonia. (See p 150.)

Suggested Reading

Arroliga AC, Podell DN, Matthay RA. Pulmonary manifestations of scleroderma. *J Thorac Imaging* 1992;7:30–45.

Asbestosis

KEY FACTS

- Asbestosis refers to pulmonary fibrosis induced by inhalation of asbestos fibers, not just asbestos exposure or asbestos-related pleural disease.

- Asbestosis typically manifests 20 to 30 years after exposure, and it is more strongly related to crocidolite than to chrysotile asbestos fiber exposure.

- Pathologically, asbestos-related pulmonary fibrosis is similar to findings in patients with other causes of UIP.

- Chest radiographs are insensitive for detecting early stages of pulmonary fibrosis. When fibrosis is sufficiently advanced to be detectable by chest radiographs, look for low lung volumes that are typically accompanied by reticular changes that predominate at the lung bases. As the fibrosis and honeycombing progresses, the classic "shaggy heart" appearance is evident.

- As with other lung fibroses, specific HRCT findings of early lung fibrosis include interlobular septal thickening, ill-defined, subpleural centrilobular nodular opacities, subpleural line formation, ground glass opacities, lobular architectural distortion, and parenchymal bands. As fibrosis progresses, honeycombing, or end-stage lung fibrosis becomes evident. Asbestos-related pleural plaques may not be evident (see Chap. 22).

- Computed tomography, especially HRCT, is much more sensitive than chest radiographs in detecting early fibrosis. Also, CT scanning easily distinguishes extrapleural fat from true pleural plaques (see Chap. 22).

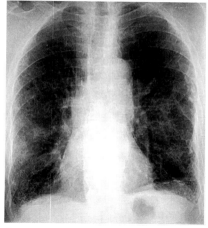

A

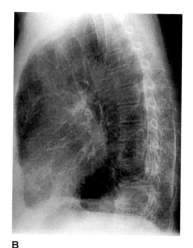

B

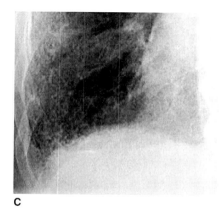

C

FIGURE 11-3

Posteroanterior **(A)** and lateral **(B)** chest radiographs of this 75-year-old man with a long history of asbestos exposure and dyspnea. Note the diffuse, coarse interstitial abnormality with lung architectural distortion typical of severe lung fibrosis. **(C)** Close-up view of the right lung base shows coarse interstitial markings with distortions of the lung architecture, typical of end-stage lung fibrosis and honeycombing. In this case the fibrosis was caused by asbestos exposure, and therefore is called asbestosis.

FIGURE 11-4

Prone high resolution CT scan shows mild lung fibrosis. Specific features in this example include ill-defined subpleural centrilobolar nodular opacities, ground glass opacities, and mild lobar architectural distortion.

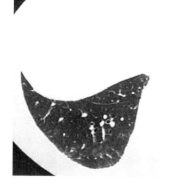
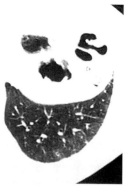

(continued)

Asbestosis (Continued)

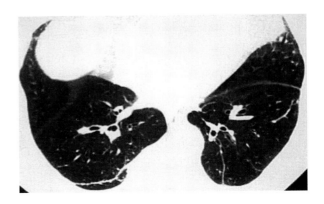

FIGURE 11-5

Prone high resolution CT scan shows mild to moderate lung fibrosis with interlobular septal thickening and parenchymal bands.

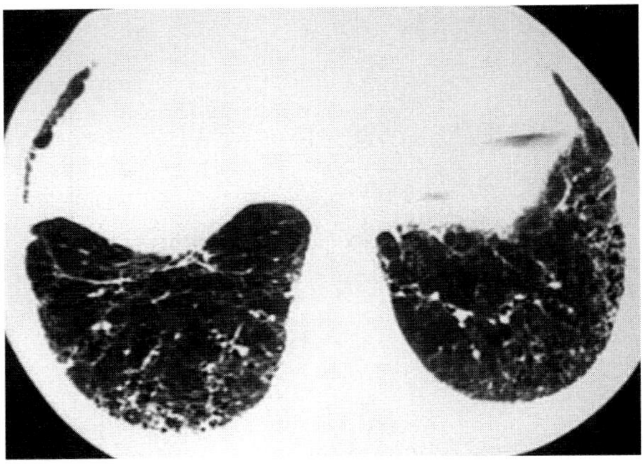

FIGURE 11-6

This HRCT scan shows early or mild honeycombing that is representative of moderately advanced lung fibrosis.

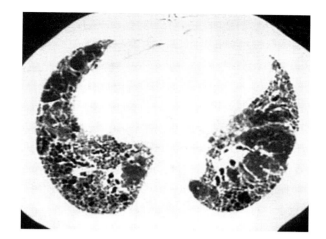

FIGURE 11-7

High resolution CT scan shows end-stage lung fibrosis and advanced honeycombing, in this case end-stage asbestosis.

Suggested Readings

Gamsu G, Aberle DR, Lynch D. Computed tomography in the diagnosis of asbestos-related thoracic disease. *J Thorac Imaging* 1989;4:61–70.

McLoud TC. Conventional radiography in the diagnosis of asbestos-related disorders. *Radiol Clin North Am* 1992;30:1177–1190.

Lymphangitic Carcinomatosis

KEY FACTS

- Lymphangitic carcinomatosis refers to spread of tumor cells into pulmonary lymphatics.
- Two mechanisms can be responsible for lymphangitic carcinomatosis. Most cases are probably caused by hematogenous spread to distal pulmonary vessels, followed by secondary invasion of lymphatics. In some instances, tumor may propagate from hilar lymphatics peripherally.
- The most common cell type to spread via the lymphatics is adenocarcinoma, which usually originates from malignancies of the lung, breast, stomach, colon, pancreas, and prostate.
- On chest radiographs, a nonspecific reticulonodular pattern is most commonly seen. The radiographic pattern is often bilateral and symmetric, unless caused by primary lung cancer, which can be unilateral.
- Bilateral pleural effusions are frequent because of lymphatic obstruction (although usually not chylous effusions). Hilar lymphadenopathy occurs in a few patients.
- Findings on HRCT scans from patients with lymphangitic carcinomatosis are both nodular and smooth interlobular septal thickening, thickened fissures (probably from subpleural lymphatic involvement), and thickening of the bronchovascular bundles. In this disease there is a combination of tumor cell infiltration and lymphatic obstruction in the interstitial space. Thickened septa are a nonspecific finding and may represent thickening by edema, cellular infiltration, or fibrosis. Lymphangitic carcinomatosis often shows a nodular or irregular thickening of the septa without the anatomic distortion of pulmonary fibrosis or the smooth thickening of edema.
- Features of sarcoidosis seen on HRCT can resemble lymphangitic carcinomatosis. In general, sarcoidosis tends to be more central, perihilar, and symmetrically bilateral in its distribution. The clinical pictures are usually quite different.
- High-resolution CT can show features of lymphangitic carcinomatosis even if the chest radiograph is interpreted as normal.

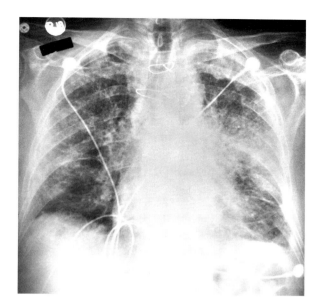

FIGURE 11-8
Posteroanterior chest radiograph shows a bilateral symmetric reticulonodular pattern caused by lymphangitic carcinomatosis in a patient with pancreatic carcinoma.

Suggested Readings

Janower ML, Blennerhassett JB. Lymphangitic spread of metastatic cancer to the lung: a radiologic-pathologic classification. *Radiology* 1971;101:267–273.

Johkoh T, Ikezoe J, Tomiyama N, et al. CT findings in lymphangitis carcinomatosis of the lung: correlation with histologic findings and pulmonary function tests. *AJR* 1992;158: 1217–1222.

Interstitial Pulmonary Edema

KEY FACTS

- Interstitial pulmonary edema is typically caused by conditions that elevate pulmonary hydrostatic pressure, acutely or chronically.

- Common causes of interstitial pulmonary edema include congestive left-sided heart failure, volume overload, and renal failure.

- Interstitial pulmonary edema is often a precursor to alveolar pulmonary edema and the two can coexist.

- Radiographic findings include a reticular pattern caused by thickened septal (Kerley's) lines, thickening and indistinctness of bronchial walls, and subpleural pulmonary edema, best seen as thickened interlobar fissures, on the lateral view. The cardiac silhouette is frequently enlarged.

- Septal lines may radiate outward from the hilum (Kerley's A lines) or arise peripherally (Kerley's B lines) in a perpendicular orientation to the chest wall in the lower lungs on posteroanterior radiographs or retrosternal region on lateral radiographs.

- Thickening of the bronchial walls is nonspecific. With congestive heart failure (CHF), it is caused by edema that collects in the peribronchial interstitial space. The term "peribronchial cuffing" is often used. Cuffing can also be caused by inflammation, such as is seen with bronchitis or asthma.

- Interstitial pulmonary edema can have rapid onset and resolution, or it can be chronic.

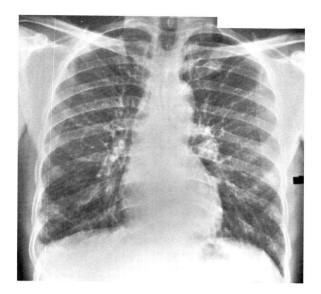

FIGURE 11-9

Posteroanterior radiograph shows a reticular pattern and mild cardiac enlargement in a patient with interstitial pulmonary edema caused by volume overload.

(continued)

Interstitial Pulmonary Edema (Continued)

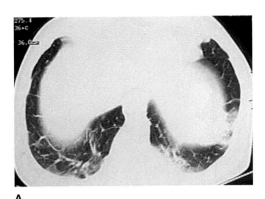
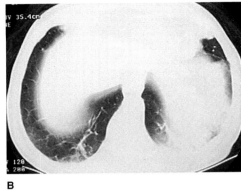

A   **B**

FIGURE 11-10   (A) Chest CT scan of a 54-year-old man with a history of congestive left heart failure shows mild thickening of the normal interlobular septa—the CT equivalent of the radiographic finding of Kerley's B lines. **(B)** Baseline CT scan from the same patient obtained before the onset of left-sided heart failure shows no evidence of interstitial pulmonary edema.

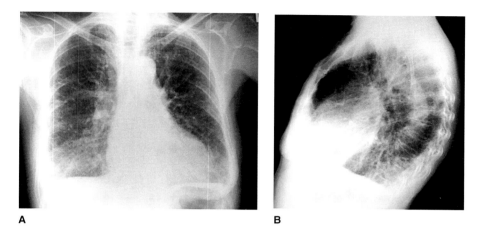

A   **B**

FIGURE 11-11   Posteroanterior **(A)** and lateral **(B)** chest radiograph of a 69-year-old-man shows cardiomegaly and prominent pulmonary interstitium resulting from chronic left-sided heart decompensation. No acute pulmonary edema is seen.

Suggested Reading

Heitzman ER, Ziter FM. Acute interstitial pulmonary edema. *Radiology* 1966;98:291–299.

Acute Respiratory Distress Syndrome

KEY FACTS

- Acute respiratory distress syndrome (ARDS) is caused by direct or indirect injury to the lung. Pathologically, it is believed to result from alveolar endothelial and epithelial injury leading to capillary leak and interstitial edema. The term "diffuse alveolar damage" is used pathologically.

- Common specific causes include sepsis, trauma, aspiration, drug use or overdose, multiple organ failure, and inhalation injury.

- The chest radiograph is often normal, as the lung injury manifests clinically during the first 24 hours.

- Ultimately, radiographs show widespread diffuse bilateral lung opacities that can be patchy.

- The heart is usually not enlarged and Kerley's lines and pleural effusions are typically absent.

- If the patient survives, radiographic abnormalities characteristically resolve very slowly over several weeks or months. Residual lung fibrosis is variable.

- Superimposed pneumonia, a common scenario, is difficult to detect or distinguish, both clinically and radiographically.

- Once a diagnosis of ARDS is made clinically, radiographs are obtained frequently to check monitoring and life support devices, as well as to detect complications such as barotrauma.

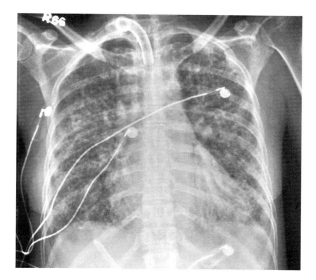

FIGURE 11-12

Supine anteroposterior chest radiograph of a 54-year-old woman who developed ARDS 3 weeks prior, as a result of a high-speed motor vehicle accident, shows diffuse, coarse lung opacities typical of severe lung injury and diffuse alveolar damage in the chronic fibroproliferative, healing phase. Note the expected position of the tracheostomy tube.

Suggested Reading

Greene R, Jantsch H, Boggis C, Strauss W. Respiratory distress with new consideration. *Radiol Clin North Am* 1983;27:699.

Pneumocystis Carinii *Pneumonia*

KEY FACTS

- *Pneumocystis carinii* pneumonia (PCP) is caused by an organism of uncertain classification (protozoan versus fungus).
- This disease is the most common human immunodeficiency virus (HIV)-related infection, although its incidence has been reduced by antibiotic prophylaxis.
- This disease typically occurs when the CD4 lymphocyte count falls below 200.
- Chest radiograph is often normal initially, although it may show a slight reduction of lung volumes as a result of "stiffer" lungs.
- A hazy "ground glass" opacity is frequently the earliest abnormality.
- Disease usually progresses to widespread parenchymal opacity, often with a perihilar distribution.
- Lung air cysts, "pneumatoceles," which occur frequently in the upper lobes, can lead to spontaneous pneumothorax, with prolonged air leak.

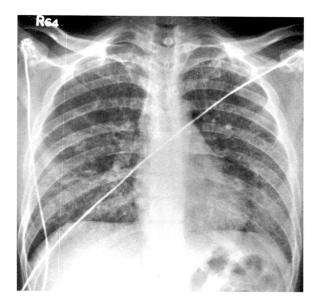

FIGURE 11-13

Anteroposterior chest radiograph of a 34-year-old man with acquired immune deficiency syndrome (AIDS) and *P. carinii* pneumonia shows diffuse, coarse interstitial opacities. This is a relatively nonspecific appearance. A suggestion of a superimposed cystic component such as often seen with *P. carinii* pneumonia is evident.

Suggested Reading

Goodman PC, Gamsu G. Pulmonary radiographic findings in the acquired immunodeficiency syndrome. *Postgrad Radiol* 1987;7:3–15.

12   Lung Cavities

Mycetoma

KEY FACTS

- Mycetomas are also called fungus balls or even aspergillomas; the most common organism involved is *Aspergillus*.
- Mycetomas represent a saprophytic collection of mycelia that develops in a preexisting space in the lung: a bulla, cavitary disease of tuberculosis, fibrobullous disease of ankylosing spondylitis, or within a cavitary neoplasm.
- The host immune system is usually normal.
- Radiographically, the mycetoma can appear to fill or nearly fill the cavity, often having a crescent of air around it; the so-called "crescent sign." Although occasionally adhered to a cavity wall, mycetomas are usually seen to fall to the dependent portion of a cavity on various decubitus views. The fungus ball often has a somewhat spongy, mottled appearance.
- Rarely, the mycetoma causes chronic inflammation of the cavity wall, lending to wall erosion and potentially massive hemoptysis. If the erosion occurs into a bronchial artery, a Rasmussen's aneurysm can form.

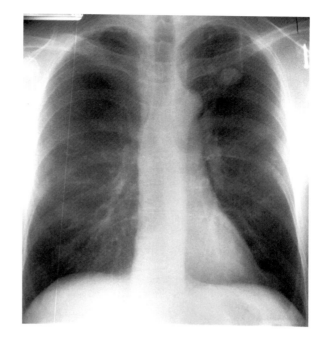

FIGURE 12-1
Posteroanterior chest radiograph of a 37-year-old-man with a prior healed pneumonia and residual left upper lobe thin-walled cavity shows a 2 cm fungus ball in a dependent portion of the cavity.

(continued)

Mycetoma (Continued)

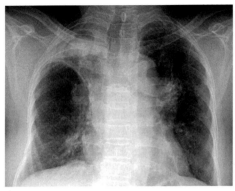

A

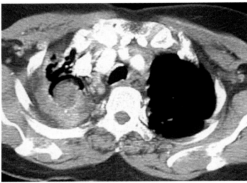

B

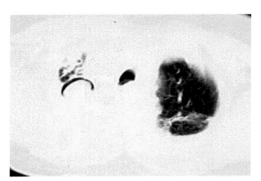

C

FIGURE 12-2

(A) Posteroanterior chest radiograph and corresponding computed tomography (CT) scans **(B)** of a 64-year-old man with a history of remote, treated, fibrocavitary tuberculosis, who presented with hemoptysis. An air-crescent is seen over a "mass" in the right upper lobe, which is classic for a mycetoma, also called a fungus ball, in an old fibrotic cavity. Note the extensive right upper lobe volume loss with elevation of the minor fissure and deviation of the trachea to the right. **(C)** CT scan also shows bronchiectasis around the cavity as part of the residual fibrotic process.

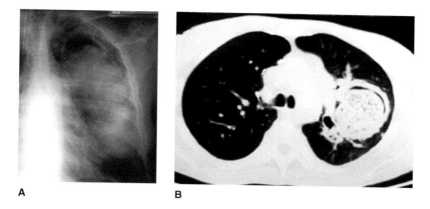

A   **B**

F I G U R E   1 2 - 3   Posteroanterior chest radiograph **(A)** and corresponding CT scan **(B)** of a 28-year-old woman with a history of treated tuberculosis shows a huge left lung mass with an air crescent, again classic for a mycetoma.

Suggested Reading

Eades KS. X-ray sign of fungal disease. *N Engl J Med* 1970;282:1216.

Pulmonary Laceration

KEY FACTS

- Pulmonary laceration implies a disruption of lung tissue causing a localized internal leak of air (pneumatocele) and blood (hematoma) in variable quantities.
- Occurs in blunt and penetrating injuries.
- Results from:
  Tearing and crushing of lung tissue from a penetrating object
     (knife, bullet, rib)
  Shearing forces and tissue stresses that occur during compression
- Usually rounded, secondary to inherent lung elasticity.
- Multiple or isolated. Multiple usually secondary to compression injuries.
- Usually 2 to 5 cm (up to 14 cm).
- Acutely, is a focal, well-circumscribed, elliptical homogeneous, soft-tissue lung mass or wedge-shaped opacity ± air-containing or air–fluid levels.
- Usually present immediately after injury but often masked by contusions.
- Can take days to form classic appearance; becomes more evident on serial examinations as contusions clear.
- Four types of lacerations have been described on the basis of CT findings and mechanism of injury:
  Compression rupture (most common)
  Compression shear (often vertical)
  Rib penetration (usually small)
  Adhesion tears (rare)

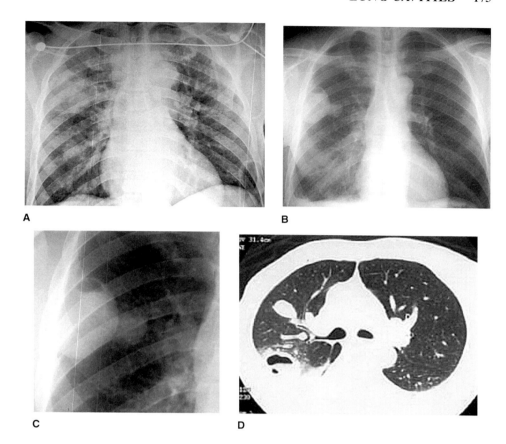

A B

C D

FIGURE 12-4 **(A)** Anteroposterior chest radiograph of a 45-year-old-man involved in a motor vehicle accident shows a nonspecific focal lung opacity in the right upper lung that is suggestive of a pulmonary contusion. **(B, C)** Posteroanterior chest radiograph obtained 4 weeks later shows two round masses in the area of previous "contusion." The larger mass has an air–fluid level. These are typical pulmonary lacerations that were initially obscured by the surrounding contusion and pulmonary hemorrhage. These are better seen in the close-up **(C)**. **(D)** CT scan confirms the intraparenchymal location of the lacerations.

Suggested Reading

Wagner RB, Crawford WO Jr, Schimpf PP. Classification of parenchymal injuries of the lung. *Radiology* 1988;167:77–82.

Pulmonary Laceration: Traumatic Pneumatocele (Stab Wound)

KEY FACTS

- The pulmonary laceration is present immediately after injury, but hemothorax or pneumothorax can obscure the underlying lung injury; the laceration becomes evident after satisfactory chest tube drainage.

- As in blunt trauma, pulmonary laceration from a stab wound can cause pulmonary hematomas, traumatic pneumatoceles, and bronchopleural fistulae.

- It can take days for the classic appearance of a traumatic pneumatocele. Look for a thin-walled, rounded lucency, usually 2 to 5 cm, depending on the size of the knife.

- If blood fills the laceration instead of air, the laceration will be more masslike (a hematoma) (see Chap. 9).

- Simple pneumatoceles heal more quickly than hematomas.

- Stab wounds do not usually have associated pulmonary contusion, whereas a gunshot wound track is surrounded by a zone of contusion of variable size.

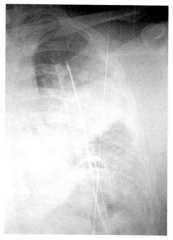

A

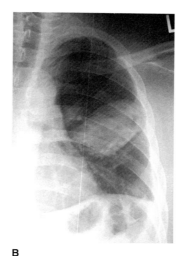

B

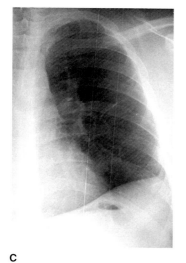

C

FIGURE 12-5

Series of chest radiographs of a 19-year-old man who suffered a stab wound to the left chest. **(A)** The immediate postoperative examination shows a dense opacification in the left midlung partially obscured by a large left hemothorax. Two thoracostomy tubes are in the expected position. The dense midlung opacification is likely a combination of a pulmonary laceration with surrounding pulmonary hemorrhage. **(B)** Two weeks after the initial injury, the pulmonary hemorrhage and pleural fluid have resolved, leaving a well-defined elliptic opacity in the left midlung, with a suggestion of some air within. This is a typical appearance for a pulmonary laceration. **(C)** Six months after the stab wound, the pulmonary laceration has healed with only a small residual scar within the lung and some blunting or scarring at the left costophrenic angle.

Suggested Reading

Groskin S. Radiological, clinical and biomechanical aspects of chest trauma. New York: Springer Verlag, 1991.

Lung Abscess

KEY FACTS

- Pyogenic pneumonias can lead to lung abscesses, which can cavitate. The most common organisms that lead to lung abscesses are *Staphylococcus aureus*, *Streptococcus pneumococcus*, and mixed anaerobic infections.

- Similar findings are noted with pulmonary septic emboli—except with septic emboli the findings are of multiple, usually smaller, lung abscesses.

- These infections can lead to simple pneumatoceles, or air cysts, as the infection clears. Pneumatoceles can resolve with little or no residua or may persist indefinitely (see Chap. 9, Multiple Septic Emboli).

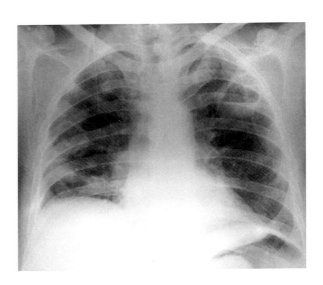

FIGURE 12-6

Anteroposterior chest radiograph of a 54-year-old-man with Staphylococcus septicemia shows multiple, peripheral lung cavities with air–fluid levels representing multiple staphylococcus abscesses, in this case from septic emboli.

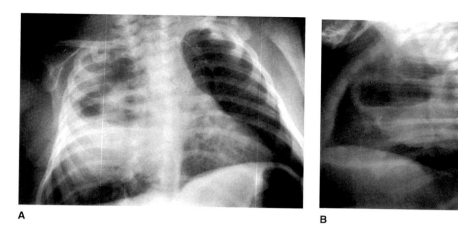

A   B

F I G U R E   1 2 - 7   Anteroposterior **(A)** and lateral **(B)** chest radiograph of a 5-month-old-child with staphylococcal pneumonia shows a large opacification with multiple air–fluid levels in the right upper lobe, representing a staphylococcal abscess.

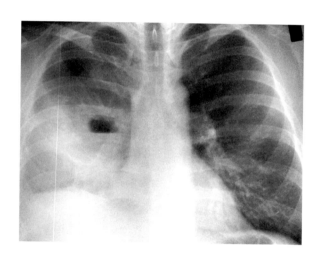

F I G U R E   1 2 - 8

Posteroanterior chest radiograph of a 30-old-man with alcoholism, poor dentition, and a mixed anaerobic flora pneumonia shows a large opacification with multiple air–fluid levels in the right upper lobe, representing a lung abscess. The superior segment of either lower lobe is a common site of aspiration.

Suggested Reading

Rubin SA, Winer-Muram HT, Ellis JV. Diagnostic imaging of pneumonia and its complications in the critically ill patients. *Clin Chest Med* 1995;16:45–59.

Parenchymal-Pleural Fistula

KEY FACTS

- A parenchymal-pleural fistula is a process, not a specific disease, in which a direct communication is seen between the pleural cavity and the lung parenchyma.

- Parenchymal-pleural fistulas remain a serious complication of a variety of lung diseases or injuries. They often necessitate operative procedures, significantly increase patient morbidity, which can prolong hospital admissions, and can have a high mortality rate.

- Parenchymal-pleural fistulas usually arise secondary to aggressive lung tumors or severe pulmonary infections such as a necrotizing pneumonia.

- Computed tomography scans show focal areas of low attenuation lung consolidation, which appears to communicate directly with an empyema, with an obvious disruption of the visceral pleura.

- Associated air in the pleural space is not necessary.

- Computed tomography scans frequently show the cause of the parenchymal-pleural fistulas. Lung cancers are well shown, as are typical findings of tuberculosis, namely marked lung destruction and scarring, with or without cavity formation.

- The relationship of a parenchymal-pleural fistula to surgical margins can be well shown with CT scanning. Associated findings of pneumonia and empyema include lung consolidation, air–fluid levels approximating the chest wall and expanding the pleural space, pleural thickening and enhancement, and the presence of loculated fluid.

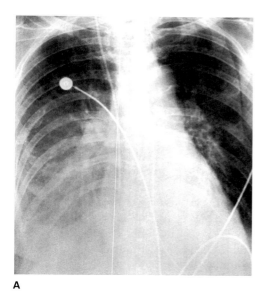

A

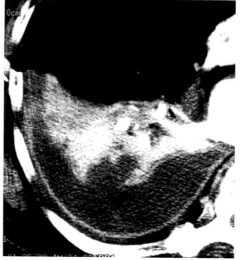

B

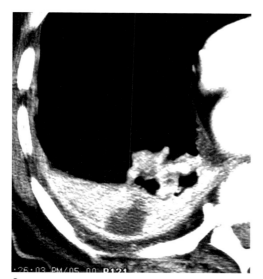

C

FIGURE 12-9

(A) An anteroposterior chest radiograph of a 74-year-old woman with type I diabetes mellitus and *Pseudomonas pneumonia* shows a right basilar lung opacity consistent with a pleural effusion; the extent of underlying atelectasis or pneumonia cannot be distinguished. **(B)** Because of persistent symptoms despite medical therapy, a contrast-enhanced CT scan obtained for further evaluation of this septic focus shows dense consolidation of the right lower lobe, consistent with pneumonia, a large pleural fluid collection, and enhanced and thickened parietal pleura, consistent with an exudative effusion. Additionally, a fluid density area is also seen within the lung consolidation, typical of a lung abscess. Note also a break in the visceral pleura, resulting in a parenchymal-pleural fistula. **(C)** Following thoracostomy tube drainage, the lung abscess or parenchymal-pleural fistula is still present; however, the pleural fluid collection is greatly reduced.

Suggested Reading

Westcott JL, Volpe JP. Peripheral bronchopleural fistula: CT evaluation in 20 patients with pneumonia, empyema, or postoperative air leak. *Radiology* 1995;196:175–181.

Echinococcus

KEY FACTS

- Most hydatid disease is caused by *Echinococcus granulosus* or *E. multilocularis*.
- Echinococcosis is endemic in sheep raising regions such as the Mediterranean, South America, and Australia. Humans are an intermediate host.
- The disease is acquired after ingestion of food contaminated by the organisms.
- The ingested ova passes to the duodenum, where larvae form, then enter the blood and are trapped by capillaries in the liver, and to a lesser extent, the lung.
- A cyst forms in the lung, which consists of an outer ectocyst and an inner endocyst. Daughter cysts attach to the endocyst. The compressed surrounding lung becomes a fibrotic pericyst.
- The typical radiographic appearance of a pulmonary echinococcal cyst is a well-defined round or oval parenchymal mass. The right lower lobe is the most common location. Cysts are multiple in one fourth of patients.
- Diameter of the cyst can range up to 20 cm. The lesion can enlarge rapidly. A doubling time of 4 months is reported.
- Rupture of the cyst allows dissection of air between the pericyst and the ectocyst, giving rise to a meniscus sign. If the cyst crumples and floats in fluid within an intact pericyst, the radiographic appearance is termed a "water-lily sign."
- Calcification of pulmonary hydatid disease is quite unusual.

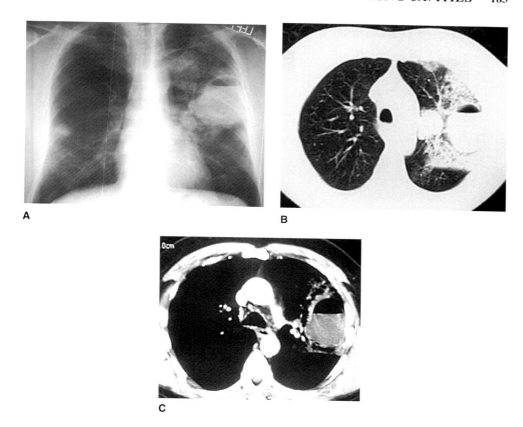

FIGURE 12-10

(A) Posteroanterior chest radiograph of a middle aged, previously healthy man with a sudden history of fever and cough shows a large fluid-filled cavity in the mid left lung. There is surrounding parenchymal opacity, another mass medially, and a second smaller focal opacity in the right lung. This subsequently proved to be caused by an *Echinococcus* infection, with sudden communication with the airways and subsequent spillage into the surrounding lung parenchyma, which explained the sudden onset of symptoms. (B, C) CT scan through the upper chest, with both lung and soft-tissue windows, again shows the large cyst in the left upper lobe, with an air–fluid level and surrounding parenchymal opacity from spillage of cystic material into the airways. A second fluid-filled cyst is seen medially. A classic water-lily sign was not evident. (Case courtesy of William Hurt, Bellevue, WA.)

Suggested Reading

Beggs I. The radiology of hydatid disease: a review. *AJR* 1985;145:639–648.

Coccidioidomycosis

KEY FACTS

- Coccidioidomycosis is caused by the fungus *Coccidioides imitis*. It is endemic to the semiarid regions of southwestern United States.
- Organisms are inhaled and form thick-walled spherules in the lungs where they incite a vigorous granulomatous response.
- Coccidioidal infection is usually self-limited but progressive disease can occur in immunocompromised patients.
- Coccidioidomycosis is classified as acute, chronic, or disseminated disease.
- Acute coccidioidomycosis manifests radiologically as segmental consolidation or multifocal nodules. One fifth of cases show adenopathy or pleural effusions.
- In chronic coccidioidomycosis, the radiograph shows persistent consolidation, which may be cavitary. The cavities can be thin or thick-walled.
- Patients with disseminated disease may have a miliary pattern on chest radiographs. The nodules can coalesce to form diffuse airspace disease.
- Calcification in coccidioidal lung nodules is rare.

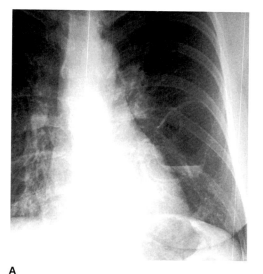

A

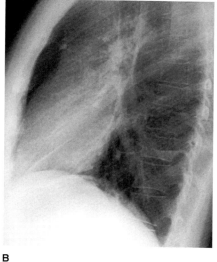

B

C

FIGURE 12-11

Posteroanterior (**A**) and lateral (**B**) chest radiograph and corresponding CT scan (**C**) of a 42-year-old woman who suffered an acute episode of coccidioidomycosis 10 years prior show two thin-walled lung cavities, both with air–fluid levels. The thin-walled cavities are the residua of the original infection. The fluid within was caused by a superinfection.

Suggested Reading

McAdams HP, Rosado-de-Christenson ML, Lesar M, et al. Thoracic mycoses from endemic fungi: radiologic-pathologic correlation. *Radiographics* 1995;15:255–270.

13 Hyperlucent Lung—Bilateral and Unilateral

Hyperlucent Lung—Bilateral

Centrilobular Emphysema

KEY FACTS

- Pulmonary emphysema, as defined by the National Heart, Lung and Blood Institute, is "an abnormal permanent enlargement of the air spaces distal to the terminal bronchioles, accompanied by destruction of the alveolar walls, and without obvious fibrosis."
- This definition excludes processes of air space dilation without alveolar wall destruction such as obstructive, compensatory, or senile hyperinflation.
- The most common form of emphysema is centrilobular; strongly associated with cigarette smoking, it results from destruction of alveoli around the proximal respiratory bronchiole with sparing of the distal alveoli.
- Centrilobular emphysema has a predilection for the upper portion of the individual lobes (e.g., the apical and posterior segments of the upper lobes and the superior segments of the lower lobes). In severe centrilobular emphysema the distal lobular alveoli may also be involved, thereby pathologically resembling panlobular emphysema.
- The accuracy of diagnosis based on chest radiographic findings depends most heavily on the severity of parenchymal destruction. With conventional radiography, the accuracy is 65% to 80%, depending on the population studied. In most patients with severe emphysema, the disease is diagnosed correctly.
- Chest radiographic features of emphysema are numerous. The most useful include flattened hemidiaphragms, paucity of peripheral vascular markings (especially in the upper lobes), and larger than expected lung volumes.
- With high resolution computed tomography (HRCT), centrilobular emphysema appears as focal areas of low-attenuation lung up to 1 cm in diameter, within a homogeneous background of normal lung parenchyma, unassociated with obvious fibrosis. Often, the centrilobular core structure is visible in the center of the emphysematous space. These areas of low attenuation are usually round or oval and have no definable wall unless partially bordered by a small vessel.

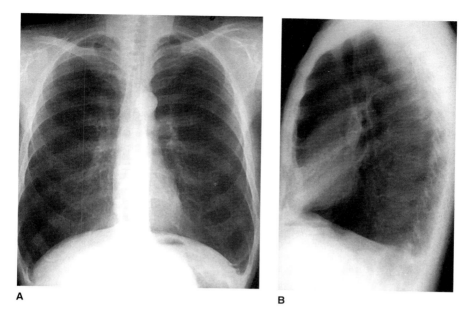

A   **B**

FIGURE 13-1   Posteroanterior **(A)** and lateral **(B)** chest radiograph of a 60-year-old man with shortness of breath and a clinical diagnosis of chronic obstructive pulmonary disease shows typical features of pulmonary emphysema: enlarged lung volumes with flattened hemidiaphragms; increased anteroposterior diameter; enlarged retrosternal space; decreased peripheral vascular markings; and a narrow, small heart.

FIGURE 13-2

High resolution CT scan of a 62-year-old man with centrilobular emphysema shows multiple focal rounded lucencies of various size (ranging from 5 to 10 mm), surrounded by normal parenchyma, without discrete walls. Note small white dots in the center of these lucencies—the preserved centrilobular core structures (*arrows*). The appearance of a partial wall may be seen when an emphysematous space abuts a vessel, usually a vein.

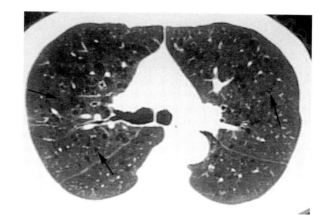

Suggested Reading

Stern EJ, Frank MS. CT of the lung in patients with pulmonary emphysema: diagnosis, quantification, and correlation with pathologic and physiologic findings. *AJR* 1994;162: 791–798.

Panlobular Emphysema

KEY FACTS

- Panlobular emphysema is a diffuse process that characteristically has a lower lobe predominance.
- Panlobular emphysema is seen most commonly in patients with alpha-1 antiprotease (antitrypsin) deficiency, but is also seen in patients with obliterative bronchiolitis, and in those abusing intravenous methylphenidate (Ritalin).
- Panlobular emphysema is seen in conjunction with smoking-related centrilobular emphysema. It is not the dominant morphologic abnormality and is probably just advanced centrilobular emphysema.
- Mild panlobular emphysema can also be a normal senescent finding in nonsmokers.

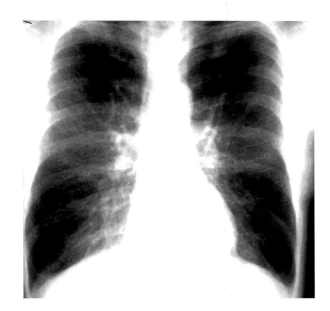

FIGURE 13-3

Posteroanterior chest radiograph of a patient with alpha-1 antiprotease deficiency shows hyperlucent lung and thinned out vascular structures at the lung periphery and bases. This appearance is typical of panlobular emphysema.

Suggested Reading

Stern EJ, Frank MS. CT of the lung in patients with pulmonary emphysema: diagnosis, quantification, and correlation with pathologic and physiologic findings. *AJR* 1994;162: 791–798.

Paraseptal Emphysema

KEY FACTS

- Paraseptal, or distal lobular, emphysema is usually a focal or multifocal abnormality involving the periphery of the pulmonary lobule, especially adjacent to connective tissue septa.

- Paraseptal emphysema is almost always seen in the periphery of the lung, including along the fissures and at sharp pleural reflections where they can appear quite cystlike. Coalescence in this type of emphysema is generally regarded as a mechanism for formation of bullae and giant bullae.

- The cause of this form of emphysema is often unknown, especially when it develops in young individuals who appear otherwise normal. It can coexist with centrilobular emphysema.

- Paraseptal emphysema appears to be important in the development of spontaneous pneumothoraces, but it is not associated with airflow obstruction. There is an increased incidence of apical bullae, formed by paraseptal emphysema, in the lungs of patients with idiopathic spontaneous pneumothorax.

- A bleb, strictly speaking, is a small vesicle—a small fluid collection—under the skin, but it can also define a form of pulmonary air cyst. The Fleischner Society has stated that a bleb of the lung is synonymous with a bulla of the lung. However, bulla, defined as a sharply demarcated area of emphysema more than 1 cm in diameter and with a wall less than 1 mm thick, is the preferred term.

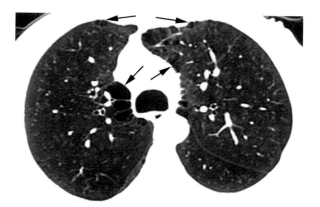

FIGURE 13-4

High resolution computed tomography (CT) scan shows paraseptal emphysema. Note the small lucencies (usually < 1 cm) that occupy a subpleural location (*arrows*). These are typical of paraseptal emphysema and should not be confused with a cystic lung disease.

Suggested Reading

Stern EJ, Frank MS. CT of the lung in patients with pulmonary emphysema: diagnosis, quantification, and correlation with pathologic and physiologic findings. *AJR* 1994;162: 791–798.

Idiopathic Giant Bullous Emphysema

KEY FACTS

- Idiopathic giant bullous emphysema is also called "vanishing lung syndrome."

- Idiopathic giant bullous emphysema is a severe, precocious, giant bullous emphysema in the upper lobes, often asymmetric, found in cigarette smoking, young dyspneic men, but can be seen in nonsmokers.

- High resolution CT shows extensive paraseptal emphysema coalescing into the giant bullae. The radiographic criteria for vanishing lung include the presence of giant bullae in one or both upper lobes, occupying at least one third of the hemithorax, usually compressing surrounding normal lung parenchyma. Seen are multiple large bullae; they vary in size from 1 to 20 cm in diameter, but are usually between 2 and 8 cm in diameter, without a single dominant giant bulla. Bullae are frequently asymmetric.

- High resolution CT can be used to distinguish among the different forms of emphysema (e.g., paraseptal emphysema and centrilobular emphysema) and to characterize the nonbullous lung by showing the extent, type, and distribution of underlying abnormalities, which may assist operative planning.

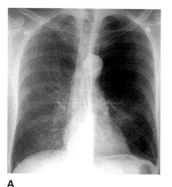

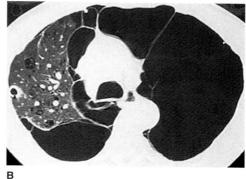

A B

FIGURE 13-5 **(A)** Posteroanterior chest radiograph of a young patient with giant bullous emphysema shows near complete absence of lung markings of the left lung, easily confused with a pneumothorax. Evidence of bulla is also seen in the right upper lobe. **(B)** HRCT chest scan shows large, bilateral, asymmetric giant upper lobe bulla. A chest tube is located peripherally in the right pleural space. No left pneumothorax is seen.

Suggested Reading

Stern EJ, Webb WR, Weinacker A, Müller NL. Idiopathic giant bullous emphysema (vanishing lung syndrome): imaging findings in nine patients. *AJR* 1994;162:279–282.

Hyperlucent Lung—Unilateral

Mastectomy

KEY FACTS

- Unilateral hyperlucent lung must be distinguished from contralateral hyperdense lung.
- When diagnosing the cause of unilateral hyperlucency, it is important to consider extrapulmonary causes such as technical factors (e.g., patient rotation) and abnormalities of the chest wall.
- Unilateral mastectomy is the most frequent nontechnical cause of a unilateral hyperlucent lung.
- Relative hyperlucency is particularly noticeable over the lower chest. It is more obvious for right mastectomies because of the summation of the cardiac silhouette and remaining breast on the contralateral side.
- Surgical clips in the axilla from lymph node dissection are useful ancillary findings of mastectomy when present.
- Unlike patients with unilateral hyperlucency from pulmonary causes, patients with unilateral mastectomy have symmetric pulmonary vasculature distribution.
- Poland's Syndrome can cause congenital unilateral absence of the breast (see Poland's Syndrome, below).

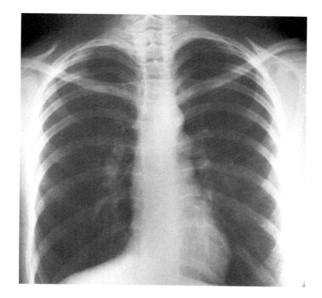

FIGURE 13-6

Posteroanterior chest radiograph of a 50-year-old woman who has had a right modified radical mastectomy for breast carcinoma. Note the relatively lucent right lung compared with the left on which the left breast and pectoral musculature are superimposed.

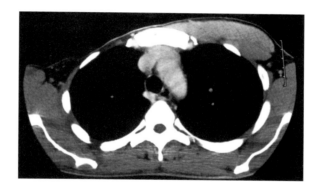

FIGURE 13-7

Chest CT scan of a 58-year-old woman who has had a right radical mastectomy for breast carcinoma. Note the complete absence of the right breast and pectoral musculature.

Suggested Reading

Culiner MM. The hyperlucent lung, a problem in differential diagnosis. *Diseases of the Chest* 1966;49:578–586.

Swyer-James Syndrome (Postinfectious Bronchiolitis Obliterans)

KEY FACTS

- Swyer-James syndrome is usually the result of a severe childhood pneumonia. Adenovirus has been implicated most widely but other causes include mycoplasma, pertussis, and measles.

- Pathologically, the condition is characterized by bronchiolitis obliterans.

- Classically, chest radiographs show unilateral hyperlucent lung, a small or normal hemithorax, a diminutive pulmonary hilum, and decrease in peripheral pulmonary artery sizes. CT scanning shows that the disease process can involve parts of both lungs or remain confined to a part of one lung. CT scans show more extensive changes than the chest radiographs, and often reveal a patchier distribution of the disease. Localized low-attenuation areas are caused by air trapping and they are accentuated by or only seen with CT scans obtained at end-exhalation.

- Patients are often asymptomatic, and the abnormality can be an incidental finding on chest radiographs or CT scanning.

- Ventilation-perfusion scanning shows decreased perfusion and retention of inhaled radionuclide on the affected side.

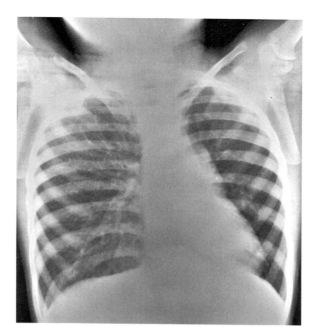

FIGURE 13-8
Posteroanterior chest radiograph from a young patient with Swyer-James syndrome shows a small hyperlucent left lung with a slight shift of the mediastinum to the left.

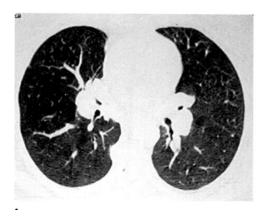

A

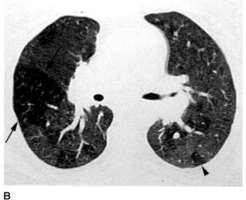

B

FIGURE 13-9 Inspiration and expiration CT scans through the midlung of a patient with postinfectious bronchiolitis obliterans show near normal parenchyma on the inspiration image **(A)** and bilateral, asymmetric multifocal air-trapping **(B)** (between the *arrows* and the *arrowhead*), typical for postinfectious obliterative bronchiolitis. A reactive small airways diseaselike asthma can have a similar appearance.

Suggested Reading

Marti-Bonmati L, Perales FR, Catala F, et al. CT findings in Swyer-James syndrome. *Radiology* 1989;172:477–480.

Tension Pneumothorax

KEY FACTS

- Pneumothorax is categorized as spontaneous or post-traumatic.
- Spontaneous pneumothorax can be further classified as primary (no apparent underlying cause) or secondary (preexisting pulmonary disease).
- Tension pneumothorax occurs when sufficient pleural air accumulates to compress the adjacent lung and mediastinum. Positive intrapleural pressure prevents proper inflation of the ipsilateral lung leading to ventilation-perfusion mismatch and decreased systemic venous return, all of which eventually result in severe cardiorespiratory compromise.
- Tension pneumothorax is most common in mechanically ventilated patients.
- Tension pneumothorax is not a radiographic diagnosis, but rather a clinical diagnosis that is only suggested by radiographs.
- Chest radiographs show ipsilateral lung compression, contralateral mediastinal shift, and ipsilateral diaphragm depression. The ipsilateral heart border may be flattened.
- Tension pneumothorax should be treated emergently with pleural drainage.

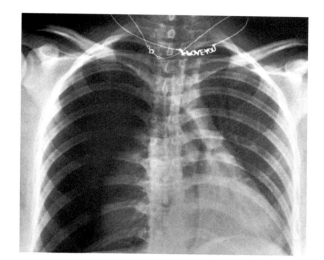

FIGURE 13-10

Upright posteroanterior chest radiograph shows a large right pneumothorax in a patient who suffered a knife wound to the right chest. Note the leftward shift of the mediastinum and depression of the right diaphragm. This appearance is strongly suggestive of, but not diagnostic of, a tension pneumothorax.

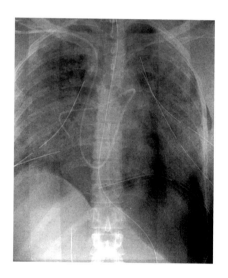

FIGURE 13-11

Supine anteroposterior chest radiograph of a mechanically ventilated patient shows a marked lucency at the left lung base, with deepening of the lateral costophrenic sulcus, the so-called "deep sulcus sign" of a basilar pneumothorax. Note the shift of the mediastinum to the right, despite several left thoracostomy tubes. In supine-positioned patients, free pleura air collects in the highest most portion of the pleural space, which is the anterior–inferior hemithorax.

Suggested Reading

Greene R, McLoud TC, Stark P. Pneumothorax. *Semin Roentgenol* 1977;12:313–325.

Pleural Effusion

KEY FACTS

- Pleural effusions are caused by excess formation or insufficient clearance of pleural fluid.
- A unilateral pleural effusion is not rare; it can result from any infectious, neoplastic, or traumatic cause.
- In addition, certain less focal diseases such as congestive heart failure and Meig's syndrome (ovarian fibroma, ascites, hydrothorax) tend to produce right-sided pleural effusions, which can be unilateral.
- Unilateral left-sided pleural effusions can be caused by esophageal perforation, pancreatitis, or aortic dissection.
- A large unilateral effusion can cause complete opacification of the hemithorax. Contralateral shift of the airway and mediastinum is the most useful method to distinguish massive effusion from unilateral lung atelectasis, which causes complete atelectasis but ipsilateral mediastinal shift.
- In a supine projection, a small or moderate unilateral effusion can layer out in the posterior pleural space causing ipsilateral haziness. In this case, the contralateral lung can appear hyperlucent.

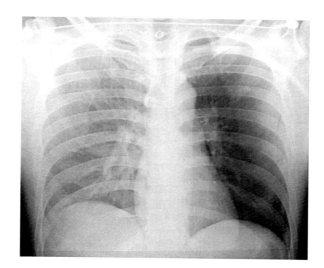

FIGURE 13-12

Supine anteroposterior chest radiograph of a 28-year-old man shows asymmetric lung opacity with the right hemithorax more opaque than the left. Alternatively, the left hemithorax can be viewed as more lucent than the right. In this case, a 600 mL right pleural effusion was found.

Suggested Reading

Woodring JH. Recognition of pleural effusion on supine radiographs. How much fluid is required? *AJR* 1984;142:59.

Poland's Syndrome

KEY FACTS

- Poland's syndrome is unilateral hypoplasia or aplasia of the pectoralis major muscle, commonly associated with ipsilateral syndactyly. Other associations include a hypoplastic forearm, microdactyly, absence of middle phalanges, aplasia of the pectoralis minor muscle, absence of one or more upper ribs on the affected side, and ipsilateral absence of the breast.
- Chest radiograph shows hyperlucency of the affected side because of the deficient chest wall musculature.
- Computed tomography scans show deficient or absent pectoralis muscle and/or breast tissue.
- Poland's syndrome must be distinguished from radical mastectomy and from surgical removal of the pectoralis musculature in patients who have undergone radical neck dissection or other procedures that require a pectoral flap.

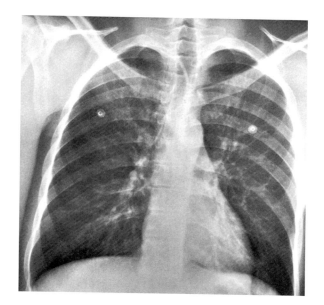

FIGURE 13-13
Posteroanterior chest radiograph shows hyperlucency of the right lung caused by the congenital absence of the pectoralis major muscle (Poland's syndrome).

Suggested Reading

Pearl M, Chow TF, Friedman E. Poland's syndrome. *Radiology* 1976;101:619–623.

Foreign Body Aspiration

K E Y   F A C T S

- Foreign body aspiration leading to a unilateral hyperlucent lung usually occurs in early childhood, especially in children aged between 1 and 3 years. Typically, it is caused by inhalation of food, especially peanuts, or toys.
- Most foreign bodies lodge in the main bronchi, occurring with approximately equal incidence.
- Persistent wheezing and cough following a choking episode are the most common presenting symptoms.
- Foreign body aspiration is most often diagnosed within days of occurrence, but can be delayed for weeks or months.
- Air trapping with a hyperlucent lung is a common manifestation of foreign body aspiration in children, whereas pneumonia and atelectasis are more common in adults. The chest radiograph may also be normal; not all foreign bodies aspirations are radiopaque.
- Paired inspiration/expiration or lateral decubitus chest radiographs are often useful to document air trapping.

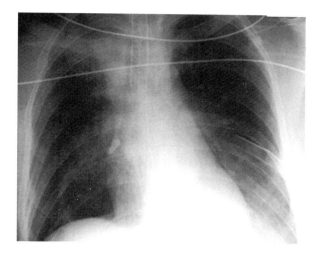

FIGURE 13-14

Anteroposterior chest radiograph of a multitrauma victim shows a molar in the right mainstem bronchus, in this case, not causing air trapping.

Suggested Reading

Strife JL. Upper airway and tracheal obstruction in infants and children. *Radiol Clin North Am* 1988;26:309–322.

Single Lung Transplantation

KEY FACTS

- Lung transplantation is an accepted and increasingly common treatment for end-stage lung disease. Specific entities treated with single lung transplantation include emphysema, cystic fibrosis, pulmonary hypertension, and a variety of interstitial lung diseases including idiopathic pulmonary fibrosis, scleroderma, and sarcoidosis.

- Bilateral lung or heart–lung transplantation is typically done for patients with cystic fibrosis and other end-stage suppurative lung disease and sometimes for other causes, such as pulmonary hypertension.

- Unilateral lung transplantation is often used for emphysema, pulmonary hypertension, and interstitial lung disease.

- Chest radiographs of patients with emphysema or pulmonary hypertension who have unilateral lung transplantation may show hyperlucency of the native lung, causing mediastinal shift and compression of the transplanted lung.

- In some cases, evidence of surgery is minimal or absent and the radiographic findings can be confusing.

- Patients with end-stage lung fibrosis who have unilateral lung transplantation may show hyperluncency of the transplant lung causing mediastinal shift toward the native lung.

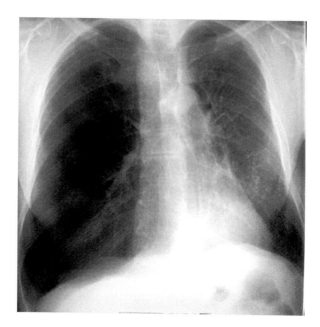

FIGURE 13-15
Posteroanterior chest radiograph of a 59-year-old man with end-stage pulmonary emphysema who received a left lung transplant shows the hyperinflated, emphysematous native right lung and the otherwise normal transplanted left lung, producing a unilateral hyperlucent lung.

Suggested Reading

Herman SJ, Rappaport DC, Weisbrod GI, et al. Single-lung transplantation: imaging features. *Radiology* 1989;170:89–93.

Pulmonary Embolism

KEY FACTS

- Pulmonary embolism causes as many as one sixth of the deaths of hospitalized patients.
- Pulmonary embolism is caused by dislodgement of thrombus that forms in the systemic veins or right atrium to the pulmonary arterial bed.
- The chest radiograph is typically the first imaging study obtained, but it is neither sensitive nor specific for the diagnosis. In the largest study, sensitivity and specificity were 33% and 59%, respectively.
- The most common chest radiographic finding is a normal examination or simply subsegmental atelectasis. Pleural effusions occur in up to one half of patients and they may be hemorrhagic. All of these findings are nonspecific.
- Much less commonly, oligemia of the lung distal to the occluded segment (Westermark's sign) can cause a unilateral hyperlucent region of the lung if the occluded segment is sufficiently large. Unilateral enlargement of a main pulmonary artery may also be seen.
- Patients in whom pulmonary infarction occurs (< 15% of pulmonary embolism) may show subpleural areas of dense opacification. Hampton's hump is a pleural-based rounded opacity caused by an infarction that typically occurs in the lower lobes (see Chap. 6).
- Infarct is uncommon because of the dual blood supply of the lung (pulmonary arterial and bronchial). Infarcts, therefore, occur more commonly in patients with impairment of the bronchial circulation (e.g., patients with congestive heart failure).
- Ventilation-perfusion scintigraphy is currently used in many institutions to stratify patients to their likelihood of pulmonary embolism. Pulmonary angiography is currently the definitive examination to identify emboli. However, spiral CT has shown promise in diagnosing central emboli noninvasively, and it may some day supplant V/Q scanning.

Suggested Reading

Buchner CB, Walker CW, Purnell GL. Pulmonary embolism: chest radiographic abnormalities. *J Thorac Imaging* 1989;4:23–27.

Endobronchial Mass

KEY FACTS

- A mass that occludes a main bronchus can cause a unilateral hyperlucent lung.

- The cause of the lucent lung is obstructive hyperinflation, whereby a check-valve mechanism allows air to enter the lung during inspiration but obstructs outflow during expiration.

- Lung cancer is the most common endobronchial mass to cause obstructive hyperinflation, yet this is a rare manifestation of central lung tumors. Atelectasis is a far more common occurrence.

- In addition to primary lung cancers, consider as relatively common causes, carcinoid tumors and airway metastases from primary skin, renal, breast, or colon cancers. Other rare benign tumors can also cause endobronchial occlusion (e.g., a chondroma).

- On the chest radiograph the central lesion is often not apparent and CT may be required to diagnose the obstructing lesion.

- An endobronchial mass can produce alveolar hypoventilation and reflex vasoconstriction, causing oligemia and a hyperlucent lung by that mechanism.

Suggested Reading

Woodring JH. Pitfalls in the diagnosis of lung cancer. *AJR* 1990;154:1165–1175.

Section 3
THE MEDIASTINUM

14   Anterior Mediastinal Masses

Thymoma

KEY FACTS

- The classic differential diagnosis for an anterior mediastinal mass involves the 4 Ts:
  Thymoma
  Thyroid goiter
  Teratoma
  Terrible lymphoma (or **T**homas Hodgkin's lymphoma)

- The most common malignant masses are metastatic adenopathy and lymphoma. Equally as common is inflammatory adenopathy secondary to sarcoidosis, infectious mononucleosis, tuberculosis, and acquired immune deficiency syndrome (AIDS).

- Other less common causes include any of the mesenchymal benign or malignant tumors that can arise from any of the normal tissues of the mediastinum, for example:
  Lymphatics → lymphangioma/lymphangiosarcoma
  Nerves → neuroma
  Artery → angiosarcoma
  Fat → lipoma/liposarcoma

- The thymus normally begins to atrophy after puberty. With computed tomography (CT) scanning, little residual thymus tissue is seen after the age of 30.

- Not all thymus enlargement is caused by a thymoma. The thymus can also be enlarged from hyperplasia, thymic cysts, thymic carcinomas, and thymolipomas.

- Thymomas account for about 10% of primary mediastinal masses. The mean patient age of presentation is 50 years.

- Thymomas are characterized as not "benign" or "malignant." They are noninvasive or invasive. One third of thymomas are invasive (and one third have myasthenia gravis, but not necessarily the same one third). After surgical resection, these tumors tend to recur locally; however, drop metastases can occur in the pleural space, even years after surgical resection.

- Noninvasive thymomas can be difficult to distinguish radiographically from invasive thymomas. With CT scanning, look for extracapsular invasion into the mediastinum. It is usually the surgeon who best defines the invasive (malignant) nature of these tumors.

- Myasthenia gravis is an autoimmune neuromuscular disorder characterized by circulating antibodies to acetylcholine receptors, leading to skeletal muscle weakness and fatigability. It is found in one third of patients with thymomas, but only about 10% of patients with myasthenia gravis have thymomas. It is much more common for these patients to have thymic lymphoid hyperplasia.

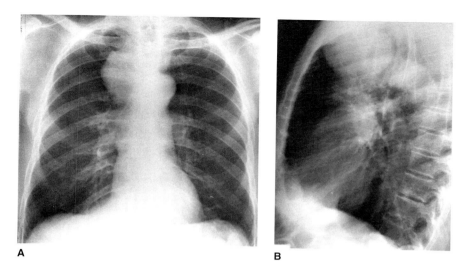

FIGURE 14-1 Posteroanterior **(A)** and lateral **(B)** chest radiograph of a 54-year-old man shows a superior and anterior mediastinal mass. This thymoma had invaded the innominate veins and artery and was unresectable.

(continued)

Thymoma (Continued)

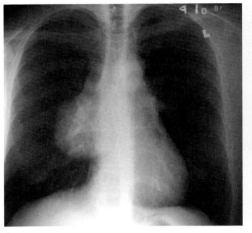 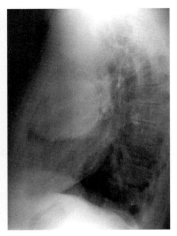

A   B

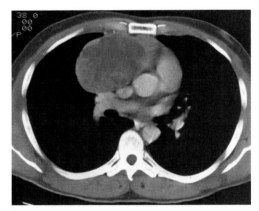

C

FIGURE 14-2

Posteroanterior (**A**) and lateral (**B**) chest radiograph of a 42-year-old man with surgically proved invasive thymoma shows a superior and anterior mediastinal mass. (**C**) CT scan shows a large heterogeneous mass in the anterior mediastinum displacing the vascular structures posteriorly. Extracapsular extension was not apparent.

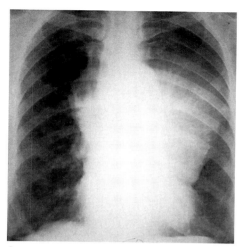
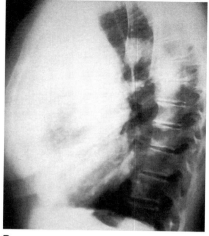

A   **B**

F I G U R E   1 4 - 3   Posteroanterior **(A)** and lateral **(B)** chest radiograph of a middle-aged asymptomatic man shows a large opacity filling the retrosternal space and silhouetting both the right and left hilar/mediastinal contours. This is a typical appearance for a large anterior mediastinal mass, in this case, a benign lipoma.

(continued)

Thymoma (Continued)

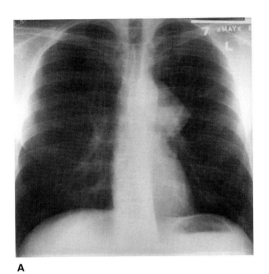

A

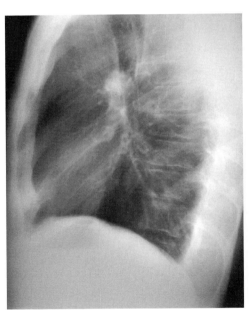

B

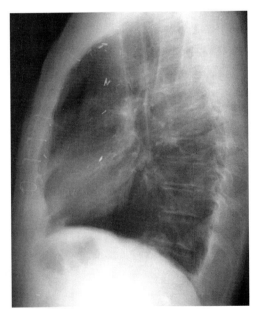

C

FIGURE 14-4
Posteroanterior (**A**) and lateral (**B**) chest radiograph of a 38-year-old man shows a superior and anterior mediastinal mass, not well seen on the lateral view. (**C**) Eight years after surgical resection of a thymoma, the tumor metastasized to the pleura covering the left hemidiaphragm; this is the so-called "drop metastasis."

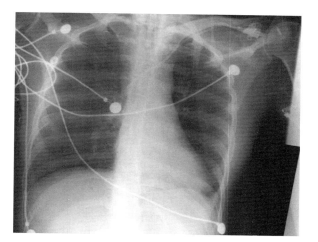

FIGURE 14-5

Anteroposterior chest radiograph of an intubated 34-year-old woman with myasthenia gravis and respiratory muscle failure shows the convexity and mild widening of the superior mediastinal contours—evidence of a thymoma. Note the soft-tissue wasting of the chest wall and shoulder musculature from the myasthenia.

Suggested Reading

Tecce PM, Fishman EK, Kuhlman JE. CT evaluation of the anterior mediastinum: spectrum of disease. *Radiographics* 1994;14:973–990.

Intrathoracic Thyroid Goiter

KEY FACTS

- A thyroid goiter can extend through the thoracic inlet into the thorax, either anterior, lateral, or posterior to the trachea. Goiters represent approximately 10% of mediastinal masses. Although mediastinal extension is usually a benign multinodular goiter, rarely a thyroid neoplasm can behave in a similar manner.

- Primary intrathoracic thyroid glands are very rare, so look for continuity with the expected position of the thyroid.

- A goiter or other enlargement of the thyroid can deviate the trachea but only rarely does it cause airway compromise.

- Always check the lateral chest radiograph for anterior or posterior tracheal deviation that may not be apparent on frontal views. The trachea should be straight and midline on both the frontal and the lateral views.

- Curvilinear calcifications around hemorrhagic cysts within the goiter may be seen on radiographs, but are best seen with CT scanning. Also on CT scanning, a goiter should show a well-defined capsule and contiguity with the cervical gland; the thyroid tissue should show some increased attenuation because of the inherent iodine content.

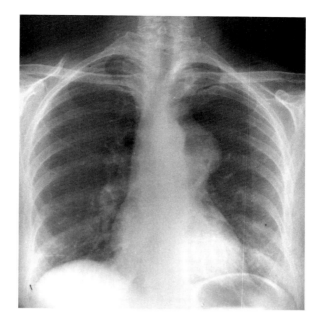

FIGURE 14-6

Posteroanterior chest radiograph of a 67-year-old man with tracheal deviation shows a superior mediastinal mass that deviates the trachea to the left; it is not clearly related to the mediastinal mass and does not silhouette the aortic arch. This was shown to be a 10 × 12 cm aberrant thyroid goiter.

(continued)

Intrathoracic Thyroid Goiter (Continued)

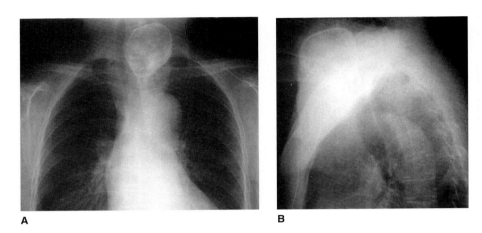

A   B

FIGURE 14-7   Posteroanterior **(A)** and lateral **(B)** chest radiograph of a 72-year-old man with a thyroid goiter shows a large calcified thyroid goiter just above the thoracic inlet.

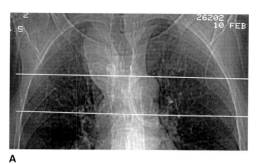
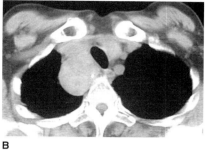

A B

FIGURE 14-8 Scout view **(A)** and a noncontrast enhanced CT scan **(B)** obtained just above the aortic arch of a 61-year-old man shows a superior mediastinal mass of relatively high attenuation, compared with muscle, typical of an intrathoracic goiter.

Suggested Reading

Glazer GM, Francis IR, Moss AA. CT diagnosis of mediastinal thyroid. *AJR* 1982;138: 495–498.

Teratoma

KEY FACTS

- Teratomas (benign, mature germ cell neoplasms) are masses derived from aberrant germ cell rests from more than one embryonic germ cell layer.

- Mature teratomas, the most common type, primarily consist of ectodermal tissues such as hair, fat, and calcium. Occasionally, enteric or pancreatic tissue is present.

- Clinically, teratomas can cause chest pain, dyspnea, and cough—occasionally trichoptysis (coughing up hair).

- Most teratomas are benign, sharply defined round or lobulated anterior mediastinal masses that present in people aged less than 30 years, but can be seen in all age groups, with a slight female predilection.

- Approximately 10% to 20% of teratomas undergo malignant transformation, in which malignant cells, particularly adenocarcinomas, are present. This is much more common in men. The mediastinum is the most common extragonadal site for these germ cell neoplasms, which include seminoma, embryonal cell carcinoma, choriocarcinoma (more common in men), yolk sac tumors, and mixed histology tumors.

- Radiographically, most teratomas occur in the anterior mediastinum. Most benign lesions are round and smooth. Teratomas can grow to 10 cm or more in diameter; they may show areas of calcification, teeth, or bone. A fat–fluid level is pathognomonic.

- Computed tomography scans are much more sensitive than chest radiographs in detecting the characteristic combinations of variable amounts of fat attenuation, soft-tissue attenuation, and bone density (or even teeth) within the mass. Fat is detected in up to one half of teratomas. Malignant characteristics such as invasion of adjacent structures are more easily delineated.

- Only very rarely does a mature teratoma undergo malignant transformation into a squamous cell carcinoma or chondrosarcoma.

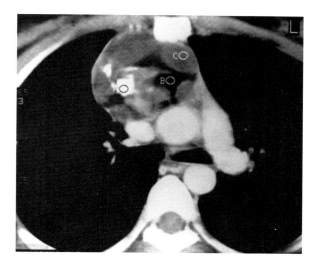

FIGURE 14-9

Computed tomography scan through the midchest of a 33-year-old woman shows an anterior mediastinal mass that has calcified, soft-tissue, and fatty components, which are typical for a benign, mature teratoma.

Suggested Reading

Rosado-de-Christenson ML, Templeton PA, Moran CA. Mediastinal germ cell tumors: radiologic and pathologic correlation. *Radiographics* 1992;12:1013–1030.

Lymphoma

KEY FACTS

- Hodgkin's lymphoma is the most frequent cancer of young adults and the most frequent lymphoma of the mediastinum.

- An equal male to female incidence of Hodgkin's lymphoma is seen, with a bimodal age frequency: ages 20 to 30 years, and 50 to 60 years.

- Hodgkin's lymphoma can grow very rapidly and can be clinically silent until very large. It can involve multiple lymph nodes, arise out of the thymus, or be infiltrating.

- Hodgkin's lymphoma can be very difficult to distinguish radiographically from other thymomas, or other anterior mediastinal masses. Therefore, it is very important to obtain histology.

- Mediastinal adenopathy is the typical manifestation of Hodgkin's lymphoma, in a usually predictable pattern involving anterior and middle mediastinal lymph nodes, with or without hilar adenopathy. Isolated hilar adenopathy is uncommon without detectable mediastinal disease. The lung is virtually never solely involved.

- In non-Hodgkin's lymphoma, the pattern of disease is more unpredictable, and it includes direct lung extension from involved nodes, lung nodules that can cavitate, and atelectasis secondary to endobronchial obstruction.

- Although the chest radiograph should detect most intrathoracic disease, CT scanning is necessary for accurate staging and therapy, especially if radiotherapy is planned. CT better evaluates the pleura and chest wall. Magnetic resonance imaging (MRI) provides additional useful information only in selected cases.

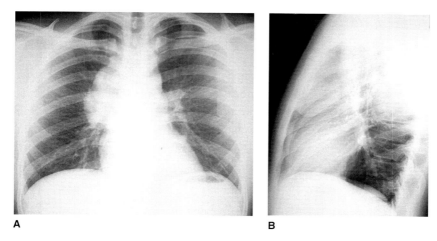

A   B

FIGURE 14-10   Posteroanterior **(A)** and lateral **(B)** chest radiograph of a 25-year-old man with vague chest pain shows a lobulated mass along the right mediastinal contour, partially obscuring the right hilum, and an opacity filling the retrosternal space, which confirms the anterior mediastinal location of this typical appearing Hodgkin's lymphoma.

Suggested Reading

North LB, Libshitz HI, Lorigan JG. Thoracic lymphoma. *Radiol Clin North Am* 1990:28; 745–762.

Castleman's Disease

KEY FACTS

- Castleman's disease, a relatively rare disorder of lymphoid tissue, is also called giant lymph node hyperplasia, angiofollicular mediastinal lymph node hyperplasia, and lymph nodal hamartoma.

- Three types of Castleman's disease are described: localized hyaline vascular (CDHV), localized plasma cell, and multicentric Castleman's disease. CDHV is by far the most common type (about 90% of cases) and is characterized histopathologically by abnormal, hypervascular lymphoid tissue.

- Most patients with Castleman's disease are young (most aged less than 30 years); no gender predilection is seen and patients are usually asymptomatic. Most of the mass lesions are found inadvertently or because of mass effect (e.g., compression of the airway).

- The lesions vary in size from 3 to 25 cm, but are usually 7 to 10 cm.

- The most common location for Castleman's disease is the mediastinum, although it occurs less commonly in the abdomen, neck, and axilla. Rare locations include larynx, vulva, pericardium, brain, subcutaneous tissue, muscle, mesentery, retroperitoneum, and pancreas.

- The radiographic findings of Castleman's disease are nonspecific. The lesions are relatively large, well-marginated masses that are sometimes lobular and may contain calcification. On CT scanning, lesions exhibit moderate to marked contrast enhancement, also a nonspecific finding.

- Although the differential diagnosis is long, lymphoma and metastatic tumors are the most important diseases to differentiate; tissue diagnosis is usually necessary. In the appropriate clinical setting, the diagnosis of Castleman's disease should be considered only after all other causes of lymphadenopathy have been excluded.

- Surgical excision is the treatment of choice for CDHV, with rare recurrence.

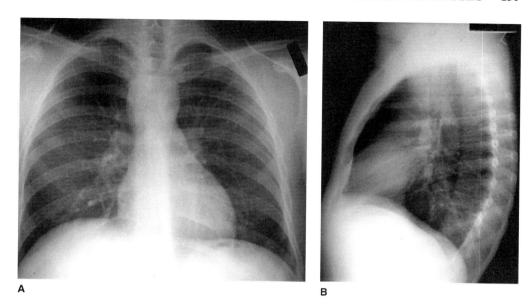

A   B

FIGURE 14-11   Posteroanterior **(A)** and lateral **(B)** chest radiographs of a 20-year-old man presenting with several months of dry cough show a smooth, well-defined, noncalcified superior mediastinal mass. This nonspecific appearance proved to be giant lymph node hyperplasia, or Castleman's disease.

Suggested Reading

Shahidi H, Myers JL, Kvale PA. Castleman's disease. *Mayo Clin Proc* 1995;70:969–977.

Mediastinal Lipomatosis

KEY FACTS

- Mediastinal lipomatosis is a condition of excess fat deposition that is usually diffusely distributed within the mediastinum.
- Conditions associated with mediastinal lipomatosis include those processes leading to central fat deposition such as exogenous steroid therapy, Cushing's disease, and generalized obesity.
- The only clinical significance is the chest radiographic confusion with other mediastinal filling or widening processes such as tumor or hematoma. The chest radiographic appearance of mediastinal lipomatosis can also mimic the saber sheath tracheal deformity (see also Chap. 16.)
- Computed tomography scanning easily distinguishes fat from other more significant abnormalities. Obviously, history and clinical presentation are also important.

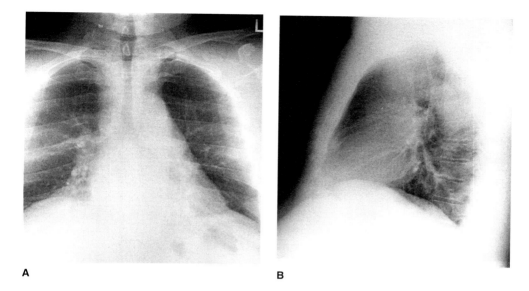

A   B

FIGURE 14-12   Posteroanterior (**A**) and lateral (**B**) chest radiographs of a 45-year-old man with mediastinal lipomatosis shows a widening of the superior mediastinum and diffuse narrowing of the trachea. This can mimic a saber sheath tracheal deformity. Also note the large body habitus and general obesity.

Suggested Reading

Homer MJ, Wechsler, RJ, Carter BL. Mediastinal lipomatosis: CT confirmation of a normal variant. *Radiology* 1978;128:657–661.

15 Middle and Posterior Mediastinal Masses

Acute Mediastinitis

KEY FACTS

- Overall incidence and prevalence of acute mediastinitis: it is unusual.
- The most common causes of mediastinitis include esophageal perforation from trauma, endoscopy, violent emesis, and postoperative infection, and esophagus rupture from a necrotic neoplasm, local extension of infection from the pharynx through the thoracic inlet.
- Patients are usually very ill with chest pain, fever, or dysphagia (with esophageal perforation). The mortality rate is high.
- In general, patients with acute mediastinitis usually show mediastinal widening with obliteration of fat planes secondary to inflammatory edema, pneumomediastinum if caused by esophageal perforation, and abscess formation with fluid collections.
- Chest radiographs can be normal or show nonspecific mediastinal widening or gas that can diffuse or is focal. In patients with postoperative mediastinitis, sternal dehiscence can be suggested by malalignment of sternal wires on the chest radiograph.
- Computed tomography (CT) scanning is useful to define the extent of mediastinitis and it may indicate its source. CT scans show increased attenuation of mediastinal fat, frank abscess (with or without air), and any fluid collections.
- In patients with esophageal perforation, esophagography is confirmatory.

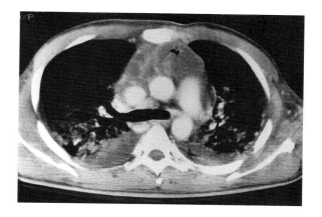

FIGURE 15-1

Computed tomography scan through the midchest of a 31-year-old man who had a severe oropharyngeal abscess shows a streaky soft-tissue attenuation (inflammation and edema) and a focal air collection (from a gas producing infection) within the normally homogeneous anterior mediastinal fat, typical for acute mediastinitis.

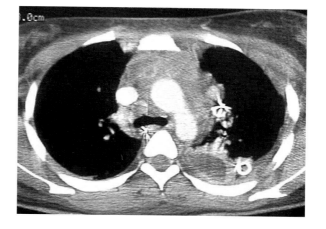

FIGURE 15-2

Computed tomography scan through the upper chest of a 17-year-old woman with acute mediastinitis following a severe dental abscess shows similar findings as in Figure 15-1, but with more extensive soft-tissue attenuation of the mediastinal fat. Also note a loculated left pleural effusion not being drained by the thoracostomy tube.

Suggested Reading

Carrol CL, Jeffrey RB, Federle MP. CT evaluation of mediastinal infection. *J Comput Assist Tomogr* 1989;11:449–454.

Histoplasmosis Mediastinitis

KEY FACTS

- Histoplasmosis is caused by *Histoplasma capsulatum*, which is found in the soil in many parts of the temperate zones of North America, especially in the Mississippi, Ohio, and St. Lawrence river valleys.

- Infection is often asymptomatic. Chest radiographic manifestations include focal parenchymal opacities and ill-defined nodular shadows. Immunocompromised patients can develop disseminated (miliary) histoplasmosis. A histoplasmoma is a nodular focus of disease, usually calcified granuloma.

- Mediastinal histoplasmosis is caused by spread of the organism from pulmonary lesions or lung parenchymal lymph nodes.

- Conglomeration of inflamed lymph nodes can lead to encroachment on mediastinal structures, especially the esophagus and airways.

- Fibrosing mediastinitis is caused by exuberant immune response to the *Histoplasma* organism and leads to dense collagen formation in the mediastinum. The chest radiograph shows widening of the mediastinum and enlarged lymph nodes that may or may not be calcified. CT scan shows the findings more clearly.

- Fibrosing mediastinitis can mimic a malignancy.

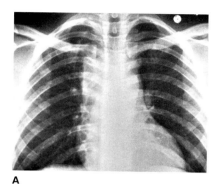

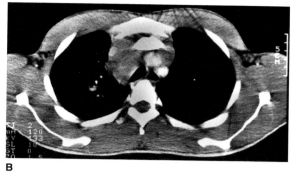

A   B

FIGURE 15-3   (**A**) Posteroanterior chest radiograph shows smooth widening of the superior mediastinum with a convex outward margin on the right side. (**B**) CT scan through the mediastinum shows a nonspecific, right-sided, soft-tissue mass displacing the great vessels, caused in this case by fibrosing mediastinitis secondary to histoplasmosis.

Suggested Reading

McAdams HP, Rosado-de-Christenson ML, Lesar M, et al. Thoracic mycoses from endemic fungi: radiologic-pathologic correlation. *Radiographics* 1995;15:255–270.

Mediastinal Small Cell Lung Cancer

KEY FACTS

- Small cell lung cancer (SCLC) accounts for 20% of bronchogenic carcinomas. It has a strong association with smoking.
- Small cell lung cancer metastasizes very early in its course. Primary lung lesion are often not evident.
- Computed tomography scanning typically shows massive hilar and mediastinal lymphadenopathy. SCLC is a common cause of the superior vena cava syndrome.
- Staging classification is different from that of nonsmall cell lung cancer. Limited disease involves ipsilateral hemithorax. Extensive disease indicates spread to the contralateral hemithorax or extrathoracic sites.
- Small cell lung cancer is not considered surgically resectable. Treatment of choice is chemotherapy. The large tumor bulk often responds dramatically to chemotherapy only to recur with a vengeance.
- Five-year survival is approximately 5%, the worst survival rate of the major bronchogenic cell types.

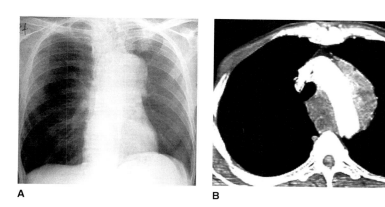

A   **B**

FIGURE 15-4   (**A**) Posteroanterior chest radiograph shows widening of the mediastinum in and around the aortic arch, which is caused by adenopathy from small cell lung cancer. (**B**) The CT scan at the level of the aortic arch better shows the extent of the tumor mass.

Suggested Reading

Rosado-de-Christenson ML, Templeton PA, Moran CA. Bronchogenic carcinoma: radiologic-pathologic correlation. *Radiographics* 1994;14:429–446.

Bronchogenic Cyst

KEY FACTS

- Foregut duplication cysts are of two types: esophogeal and bronchogenic.
- Most bronchogenic cysts are lined by pseudostratified columnar epithelium and contain cartilage.
- Approximately 75% arise in the mediastinum; the others occur within the lung parenchyma.
- On chest radiographs, most cysts are found in relation to the carina (usually subcarinal) and have a smooth contour. They may contain rim calcification or milk of calcium.
- An air–fluid level indicates communication with the tracheobronchial tree and, possibly, infection.
- On CT, the finding of a nonenhancing mass of uniform water density is confirmatory. Hemorrhage or protein can cause a higher density.
- Asymptomatic cysts can be observed, but they are often aspirated or removed surgically.
- (See also Chap. 7.)

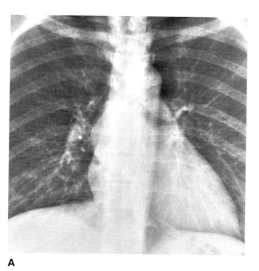

A

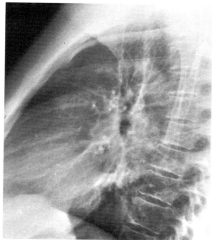

B

C

FIGURE 15-5

Posteroanterior (**A**) and lateral (**B**) chest radiographs show an ovoid pulmonary nodule in the right lower lobe, just beneath the right mainstem bronchus. (**C**) CT scan shows the homogeneous, low density character of the lesion. This is a typical intraparenchymal bronchogenic cyst.

Suggested Reading

Fitch SJ, Tonkin ILD, Tonkin AK. Imaging of foregut duplication cysts. *Radiographics* 1986; 6:189.

Neurogenic Tumor

KEY FACTS

- Neurogenic tumors are by far the most common cause of posterior mediastinal masses. Other causes include extension of other masses to the posterior mediastinum and paraspinous inflammatory processes.

- Tumors of neurogenic origin can be classified as arising from the peripheral nerves, the sympathetic ganglia, or the paraganglionic cells.

- Tumors of peripheral nerve cell origin include schwannomas, neurofibromas, and their sarcomatous counterparts.

- Peripheral nerve cell tumors are more common in patients with Von Recklinghausen's disease.

- Radiographically, these tumors are well-defined and, with intraspinal extension, they can have a dumbbell appearance. On CT, cystic areas in these tumors can cause lower than soft-tissue attenuation values.

- Tumors of the sympathetic ganglion cells include neuroblastoma, ganglioneuroblastoma, and ganglioneuroma in decreasing order of malignant behavior.

- Most of these tumors occur in children and young adults.

- Radiographically, sympathetic ganglion tumors can assume a vertical orientation similar to the sympathetic ganglion chain. Calcification is common.

- Paragangliomas are rare and include chemodectomas or pheochromocytomas. On CT, these tumors usually enhance substantially.

(continued)

Neurogenic Tumor *(Continued)*

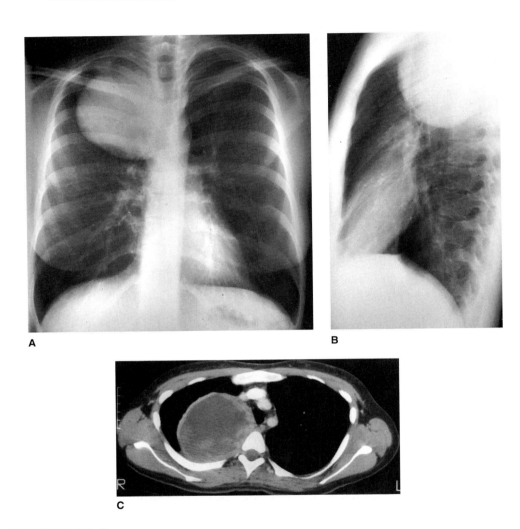

FIGURE 15-6

Posteroanterior (**A**) and lateral (**B**) chest radiographs of a 26-year-old-woman complaining of right chest pain after minor chest trauma show a large extraparenchymal mass along the right mediastinal contour, slightly displacing the trachea to the left. Although this could represent a hematoma, the clinical presentation and radiograph led to a CT scan for further evaluation. (**C**) CT scan through the mass shows a heterogeneous mass with possible extension through the neural foramina on the right.

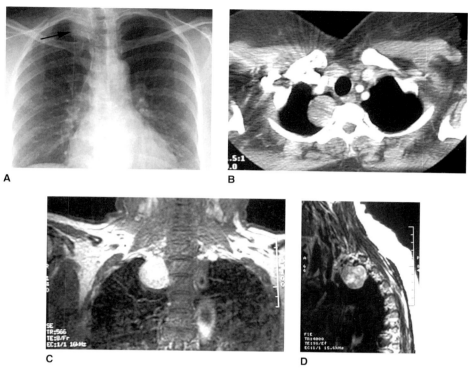

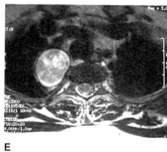

FIGURE 15-7

(**A**) Posteroanterior chest radiograph from a 37-year-old man with an incidental finding of a right apical rounded mass that appeared to be extrapleural. (**B**) CT scan through this mass shows an extravascular, homogeneously enhancing mass in a typical location for a neurogenic tumor. (**C, D, E**) Multiplanar magnetic resonance image (MRI) shows the extravascular mass to be of mixed signal intensity. No chest wall invasion or extension from a neural foramina is seen.

Suggested Reading

Reed JC, Haller KK, Feigin DS. Neural tumors of the thorax: subject review from the AFIP. *Radiology* 1978;126:9–17.

Mediastinal Lymphangioma

KEY FACTS

- Lymphangiomas are benign tumors of the lymphatic system that comprise 0.7% to 4.5% of mediastinal tumors.

- Lymphangiomas are most commonly located in the anterior or superior mediastinum.

- A male predominance is seen for this tumor, which usually is found prior to age 2 years, but the lesion may first manifest in adulthood.

- Most presentations during adulthood are asymptomatic and some reflect a recurrence from an incompletely resected childhood lesion.

- The chest radiographic appearance is that of a nonspecific mediastinal mass.

- On CT, more than half of mediastinal lymphangiomas are entirely or predominantly cystic with attenuation values slightly higher than that of water. Postcontrast enhancement is uncommon.

- The MRI appearance of lymphangioma is similar to that of CT but MRI may more clearly show the cystic components of the lesion as well as extension into the soft tissues of the neck (cystic hygroma).

- Surgery is usually recommended because these lesions tend to grow.

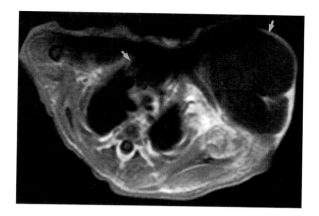

FIGURE 15-8
T1-weighted axial MRI in a young boy shows a low signal intensity lesion that involves both the left chest wall and upper anterior mediastinum (*arrows*).

Suggested Reading

Shaffer K, Rosado-de-Christenson ML, Patz EF, et al. Thoracic lymphangioma in adults: CT and MR imaging features. *AJR* 1994;162:283–289.

16 Airway Diseases

Tracheal Bronchus

KEY FACTS

- The tracheal bronchus, a rare congenital abnormality seen in 1% to 2% of bronchoscopic examinations, is a condition in which a bronchus originates directly from the tracheal wall. It occurs almost exclusively on the right side and involves predominantly the upper lobes. Two variations are known: (1) ectopia of the upper lobe apical segmental bronchus or, more rarely, (2) a true supernumerary bronchus. Three segmental bronchi should be seen in a complete right upper pulmonary lobe.

- The tracheal bronchus can be a finding on a routine chest radiograph showing a right-sided tubular lumen near the lower lateral trachea.

- Computed tomography (CT) scan of the chest shows a bronchus arising directly from the right wall of the trachea.

- Bronchoscopic examination shows an accessory bronchus opening on the tracheal wall a few centimeters above the carina.

- In many instances, a tracheal bronchus is of no clinical consequence but cases have been associated with recurrent bronchial infections, postobstructive pneumonias, bronchiectasis, congenital cystic adenomatoid malformation, difficult endotracheal intubation with intraoperative hypoxemia caused by tube obstruction of the tracheal bronchus and collapse of the right upper lobe, and localized lung cancer.

- The diagnosis of the tracheal bronchus when associated with morbidity is usually made during infancy.

- The tracheal bronchus does not usually necessitate specific treatment unless surgical excision of the involved segment is indicated for localized bronchiectasis, hemorrhage, or cancer.

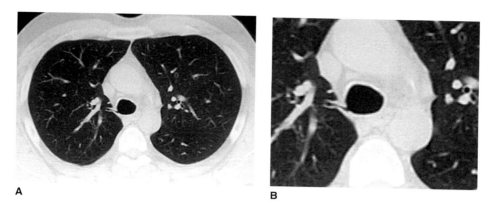

FIGURE 16-1   (A) Computed tomography scan of the chest shows a small tracheal bronchus arising directly from the right wall of the trachea. (B) Close-up view.

Suggested Reading

Freeman SJ, Harvey JE, Goddard PR. Demonstration of supernumerary tracheal bronchus by computed tomographic scanning and magnetic resonance imaging. *Thorax* 1995;50: 426–427.

Saber-Sheath Trachea

- Saber-sheath tracheal deformity is an acquired abnormality related to the pulmonary mechanics of long-standing airway obstruction and cough. Most saber-sheath tracheas occur in older men with obstructive pulmonary disease.
- Saber-sheath tracheal deformity involves only the intrathoracic trachea. The coronal diameter of the trachea is two thirds or less than is the sagittal diameter. This can be assessed either by posteroanterior and lateral chest radiographs or CT scanning. The trachea can have densely calcified cartilages.
- The cause is unknown, but it probably reflects the influence of intrathoracic transmural pressures on the tracheal wall.
- Saber-sheath tracheal deformity is the best chest radiographic sign for chronic bronchitis and chronic obstructive pulmonary disease (COPD), with a specificity of 95%, but a sensitivity of only 55%.
- Differential diagnosis includes extrinsic tracheal compression by mediastinal masses such as intrathoracic goiters or lymphomas, and mediastinal lipomatosis (see Chap. 14).

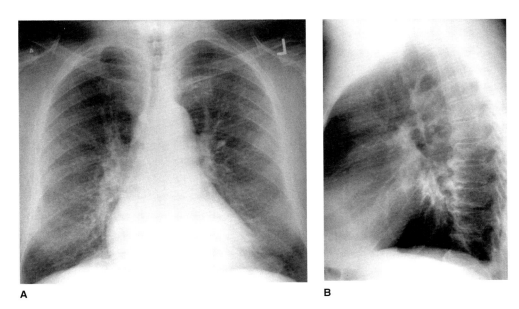

A   **B**

FIGURE 16-2   Posteroanterior (**A**) and lateral (**B**) chest radiographs of a 69-year-old-man show typical saber sheath-tracheal deformity; the intrathoracic trachea is narrowed in the frontal view of the chest and widened in the lateral view. Note the associated pulmonary emphysema.

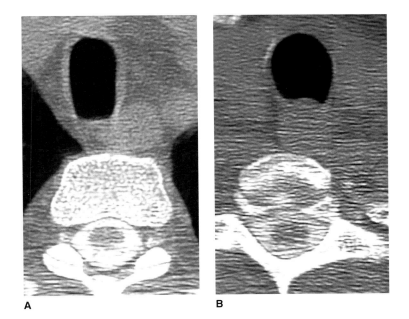

A   **B**

FIGURE 16-3   (**A**) Computed tomography scan through the intrathoracic trachea of a 55-year-old man with chronic obstructive pulmonary disease shows the typical cross-sectional appearance of the saber sheath-tracheal deformity. The coronal diameter of the trachea is less than two thirds of the sagittal diameter. Compare this shape with the normal round shape of the trachea (**B**), as seen in the same patient at an extrathoracic level, in the neck.

Suggested Reading

Greene R, Lechner GL. "Saber-sheath" trachea: a clinical and functional study of marked coronal narrowing of the intrathoracic trachea. *Radiology* 1975;115:265–268.

Tracheal Stenosis

KEY FACTS

- Tracheal stenosis commonly results from inflammatory granulomas causing localized tracheal narrowing and fixed stenosis.
- Common causes include:

   Post-traumatic or iatrogenic injury
   Tuberculosis
   Fungal infections, such as histoplasmosis
   Wegener's granulomatosis

- Less commonly, tracheal narrowing can be caused by a primary tracheal neoplasm.
- Neoplasms of adjacent structures, such as the thyroid (see Chap. 14), lung, and esophagus can invade the trachea, and may actually be the most common of the neoplastic diseases to affect it. CT is useful in ruling out external compression of the trachea by a mass or vascular anomaly.

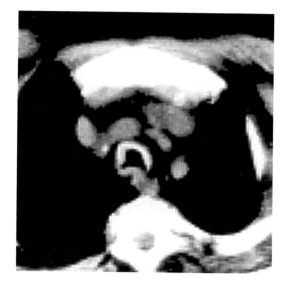

FIGURE 16-4

Computed tomography scan through the mid-trachea of a patient with tracheal stenosis secondary to Wegener's granulomatosis. The tracheal diameter is 9 mm (normal is approximately 20 mm).

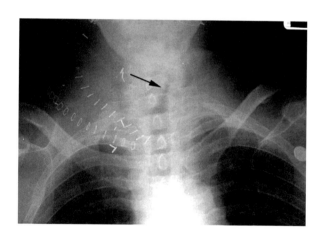

FIGURE 16-5

Anteroposterior chest radiograph of a patient who underwent recent vascular surgery of the neck shows a soft-tissue opacity overlying the right neck, deviating the trachea to the left (*arrow*), which proved to be a hematoma.

Suggested Reading

Gamsu G, Webb WR. Computed tomography of the trachea: normal and abnormal. *AJR* 1982; 139:321–326.

Tracheomalacia

KEY FACTS

- Tracheomalacia is characterized by increased tracheal compliance, which can result in a functional (i.e., not fixed) obstruction or stenosis.

- Tracheomalacia is usually focal, but it can be diffuse. Most causes are acquired; the most common is ischemic necrosis from an overinflated endotracheal tube cuff; however, the incidence of this injury has decreased with the advent of low-pressure cuffs. Other less common causes include trauma, radiation therapy, tracheoesophageal fistula and complications arising from its surgical repair, and relapsing polychondritis.

- Tracheomalacia can also develop after resection of an extrinsic mass or anomalous vessel that had compressed or displaced the airway and caused airflow obstruction to persist for months or even years after the operation.

- A CT scan obtained during suspended inspiration cannot show abnormal flaccidity of the trachea or bronchi. Tracheal collapse is most pronounced during exhalation, therefore, dynamic maneuvers must be used to show the increased compliance. In patients with tracheomalacia, expiratory CT shows tracheal collapse ranging from approximately 60% to 100% of the cross-sectional area of the trachea, from inspiration.

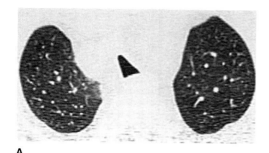

A

FIGURE 16-6

(**A, B**) Selected CT scans of the trachea of a patient with idiopathic tracheomalacia show an abnormal triangular shape to the normal, usually round cross-sectional appearance of the trachea. (**C**) Note the motion artifact (*arrows*), hence a double exposure, of the lateral tracheal walls showing the abnormal wall motion. Normally, the posterior membrane moves anterior and posterior with respiration.

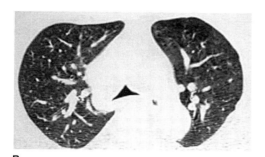

B

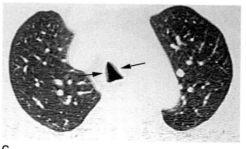

C

Suggested Reading

Frey E, Smith W, Grandgeorge S, et al. Chronic airway obstruction in children: evaluation with cine-CT. *AJR* 1987;148:347–352.

Tracheobronchopathia Osteochondroplastica

KEY FACTS

- Tracheobronchopathia osteochondroplastica is an unusual idiopathic condition in which nodules of mature bone, bone marrow, and cartilage form and protrude into the lumen of the airway, usually the trachea and main bronchi. The lesions always spare the membranous posterior wall of the trachea and main bronchi.

- Tracheobronchopathia osteochondroplastica is most common in men aged more than 50 years; it is usually asymptomatic, but can present with symptoms related to airway obstruction (e.g., expiratory wheezing and recurrent pneumonia).

- The incidence is reported as 1 of 200 in an autopsy series; 90% of cases are diagnosed at autopsy as an incidental finding.

- Tracheobronchopathia osteochondroplastica has a characteristic appearance both on CT scan and direct visualization. CT scan shows a calcified tracheal cartilaginous ring with nodular calcific protuberances that narrow the lumen. The CT scan appearance is similar to amyloidosis except the posterior membrane is spared.

- The course of tracheobronchopathia osteochondroplastica is generally indolent and it does not represent a malignant process.

- The differential diagnosis for nodular tracheal lesions includes tracheobronchopathia osteochondroplastica, tracheal amyloidosis, endobronchial sarcoidosis, and tracheal papillomatosis.

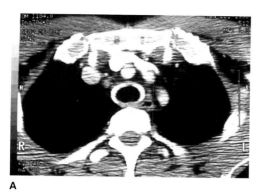
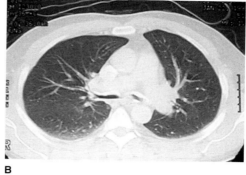

A   B

FIGURE 16-7   Selected CT scan images of a 66-year-old man being evaluated for a lung mass show dense tracheal cartilage calcification (**A**) and narrowed, calcified walls of both main bronchi (**B**), typical for tracheobronchopathia osteochondroplastica.

Suggested Reading

Prakash UBS. Tracheobronchopathia osteochondroplastica. *Ann Otol Rhinol Laryngol* 1990: 99;689–694.

Tracheal and Endobronchial Neoplasms

KEY FACTS

- Primary malignant neoplasms are uncommon, although in the adult they are slightly more common than benign primary tracheal neoplasms; they include squamous cell carcinoma, adenocarcinoma, and adenoid cystic carcinoma (mixed salivary gland tumors.)

- Carcinomas account for 60% to 90% of primary malignant tracheal neoplasms. Tracheal squamous cell carcinomas are most common in the lower one third of the trachea. Less common malignant tracheal neoplasms are chondrosarcoma, fibrous sarcoma, and carcinoid and other rare mesenchymal tumors.

- Secondary malignant neoplasms of the trachea are also unusual; they are seen in approximately 2% of patients dying from solid tumors and 5% of patients with multiple metastases. The common primary neoplasms to metastasize to the trachea are breast, colon, genitourinary tract (including testes), melanoma, and Kaposi's sarcoma. The radiographic and CT features are indistinguishable from central primary neoplasms.

- Bronchogenic carcinoma is the most important disease of the central bronchi. More than 60% of bronchogenic carcinomas arise in the lobar, segmental, or subsegmental bronchi. These tumors are most conveniently subdivided into small cell carcinoma and the non–small-cell carcinoma (adenocarcinoma, squamous carcinoma, and large-cell carcinoma). (For further discussion of lung cancer, see Chap. 8).

- Benign neoplasms of the central airways include hamartoma and squamous papilloma. The term "bronchial adenoma," which is no longer used, formerly was applied to a group of lung tumors, of which 85% were carcinoid tumors and 15% cylindromas. The problem with the term "bronchial adenoma" was that it did not reflect the heterogeneity or the malignant potential of these tumors. Despite the malignant potential, most bronchial carcinoids can be cured.

- Bronchial carcinoid tumors are usually central and can calcify when large. CT scanning shows calcification in carcinoid tumors in up to 39% of lesions; the calcifications are often large and chunky.

- Well-differentiated carcinoid tumors constitute about 90% of bronchial carcinoids, whereas atypical carcinoid tumors, which have a higher malignant potential, constitute the remaining 10%. The carcinoid syndrome is rare among cases of carcinoid tumors of the tracheobronchial tree.

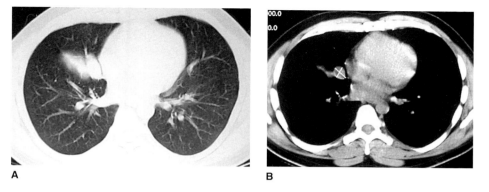

A B

FIGURE 16-8 Chest CT scans, lung (A) and soft-tissue (B) windows, of a 32-year-old man with recurrent right middle lobe pneumonia. Note the somewhat tubular soft-tissue mass at the take-off of the right middle lobe bronchus, which subsequently proved to be a carcinoid tumor. (Case courtesy of W. Caras, Tacoma, WA.)

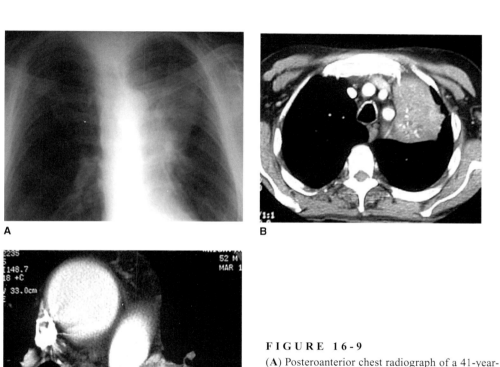

A B

C

FIGURE 16-9

(A) Posteroanterior chest radiograph of a 41-year-old man with an incidentally discovered chest abnormality after a minor traffic accident shows left upper lobe collapse. (B) CT scan through the midtrachea shows the left upper lobe collapse with a drowned lung appearance (low attenuation parenchyma, enhancing vessels and mucus bronchograms). (C) CT scan through the left main bronchus and upper lobe bronchus shows a typical large central carcinoid tumor with chunky irregular calcifications.

Suggested Reading

Mayr B, Ingrisch H, Haussinger K, et al. Tumors of the bronchi: role of evaluation with CT. *Radiology* 1989;172:647–652.

Right Pneumonectomy Syndrome

KEY FACTS

- Right pneumonectomy syndrome is a rare, delayed complication of pneumonectomy of the right lung (< 0.5%) that occurs in all ages but is most common in children and adolescents.

- During the first year after pneumonectomy, a marked right-posterior deviation of the mediastinum is seen, with counterclockwise rotation of the heart and great vessels, and displacement of the hyperinflated left lung into the right, anterior hemithorax.

- These findings are clearly shown with chest CT scans.

- Realignment of intrathoracic structures results in compression of the left main bronchus, distal trachea, or left lower lobe bronchus between the left pulmonary artery anteriorly and the aorta or thoracic spine posteriorly.

- Surgical intervention, including removal of adhesions, pericardial or intercostal flaps to stabilize the thoracic structures, and placement of various types of implants to fill the empty hemithorax, is performed to correct right pneumonectomy syndrome.

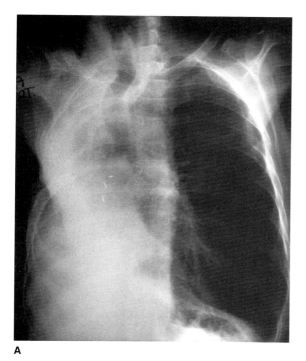

A

FIGURE 16-10

(A) Posteroanterior chest radiograph of a 63-year-old man who presented with several episodes of recurrent left lower lobe pneumonia since a right pneumonectomy for bronchogenic carcinoma 2 years prior shows the expected thoracotomy and pneumonectomy changes with complete opacification of the right hemithorax, and shift and rotation of the mediastinum to the right. Also note a hyperinflated left lung with no definite left lower lobe disease. (B) Chest CT scan performed to evaluate for recurrent tumor shows narrowing of the left lower lobe bronchus, which is squeezed between the descending thoracic aorta and the left pulmonary artery, and (C) subtending left lower lobe pneumonia.

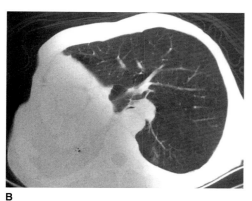

B

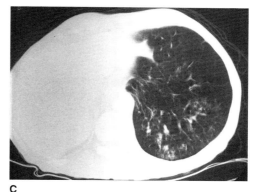

C

Suggested Reading

Shepard JA, Grillo HC, McLoud TC, et al. Right-pneumonectomy syndrome: radiologic findings and CT correlation. *Radiology* 1986;161:661-664.

Bronchiectasis

KEY FACTS

- Bronchiectasis is defined as the permanent abnormal dilation of bronchi resulting from destruction of the elastic and muscular components of the bronchial wall.
- The most common causes of bronchiectasis are:

   Necrotizing bacterial or viral infection in childhood
   Cystic fibrosis
   Other less common causes include:
   Inmotile cilia syndromes, including Kartagener's syndrome
   Allergic bronchopulmonary aspergillosis
   Immunoglobulinopathies
   Human immunodeficiency virus (HIV) infection
- Bronchiectasis is best evaluated with CT scanning, especially high resolution CT scanning.
- Computed tomography scan signs of bronchiectasis include:
   Bronchial wall thickening caused by peribronchial inflammation and fibrosis
   Dilated nontapering bronchi in the periphery of the lung
   Air–fluid levels in distended bronchi
   Linear array or cluster of cystlike spaces
- Cylindrical bronchiectasis is the least severe form.
- Varicose bronchiectasis has alternating dilation and constriction yielding a beaded, varicoid appearance.
- Saccular and cystic bronchiectasis are the most severe forms; the airways are markedly dilated.
- Patients with bronchiectasis can have concomitant severe parenchymal destruction and small airways obliterative bronchiolitis.

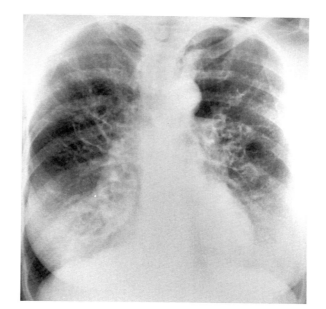

FIGURE 16-11
Posteroanterior chest radiograph of a patient with severe cystic bronchiectasis shows multiple perihilar ring shadows and tram tracking typical for bronchiectasis. In this patient, the bronchiectasis developed after a presumed viral pneumonia during childhood.

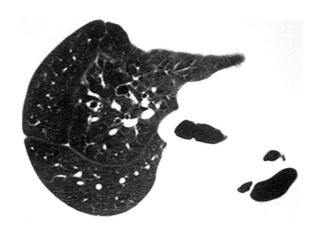

FIGURES 16-12, 16-13, and 16-14
High resolution CT scans from three different patients show the morphologic similarity and variability of bronchiectasis.

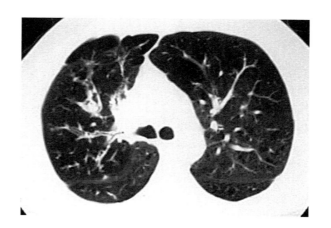

FIGURE 16-13

(continued)

Bronchiectasis (Continued)

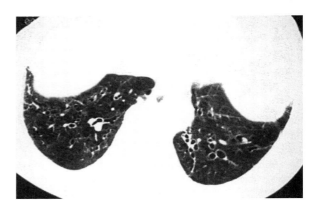

FIGURE 16-14

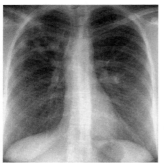

A

FIGURE 16-15

(**A**) Posteroanterior chest radiograph of a woman with a history of asthma. Note the branching tubular opacities in the right upper lobe typical of the so-called "finger-in-glove" appearance of mucus impacted bronchiectatic airways in this patient with allergic bronchopulmonary aspergillosis. (**B, C**) CT scans through the right upper lobe of this woman with allergic bronchopulmonary aspergillosis better show the bronchiectatic airways, some air-filled, others impacted with mucus.

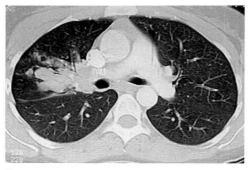

B

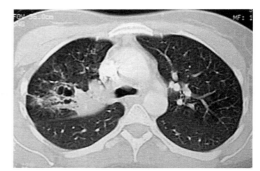

C

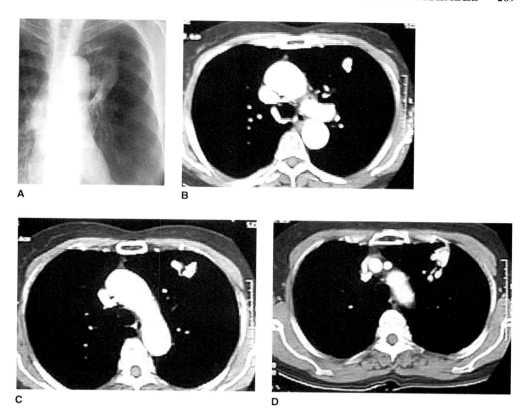

FIGURE 16-16 (**A**) Posteroanterior chest radiograph of a 71-year-old man with a history of treated tuberculosis shows a tubular mass in the left upper lobe. CT scanning showed this mass to be calcified and dividing in the cephalad direction, over serial slices. (**B**) Note the single calcified nodule, (**C**) the two calcified nodules, and (**D**) the four calcified nodules. This results from bronchiectasis that subsequently became impacted with mucus and then calcified. We like to call this a "staghorn calculus of the lung."

Suggested Reading

Müller NL, Bergin CJ, Ostrow DN, et al. Role of computed tomography in the recognition of bronchiectasis. *AJR* 1984;143:971–976.

Cystic Fibrosis

KEY FACTS

- Cystic fibrosis was first described as a separate entity in 1938. In the 1950s, it was recognized that the disease produces elevated sodium and chloride levels in sweat.

- An abnormal gene on chromosome 7 has been implicated in 70% of cases. Transmission is by autosomal recessive mode. Ninety-five percent of patients are Caucasian.

- Although most patients with cystic fibrosis are children, 7% are diagnosed at age 31 or older.

- A primary pathologic characteristic of cystic fibrosis is obstruction of small bronchi by mucus. Inspissated mucus is often colonized by *Pseudomonas* species.

- Radiographically, bronchiectasis in cystic fibrosis is often saccular. The dilated bronchi can contain air–fluid levels or mucus plugs. The lungs are hyperinflated because of air trapping.

- Superinfection can occur with *Pseudomonas* infections and also with atypical mycobacteria and allergic bronchopulmonary aspergillosis.

- Computed tomography scans show thick-walled, nontapering, dilated airways as well as small centrilobular nodules that can have a tree-in-bud appearance, corresponding to inflamed small airways.

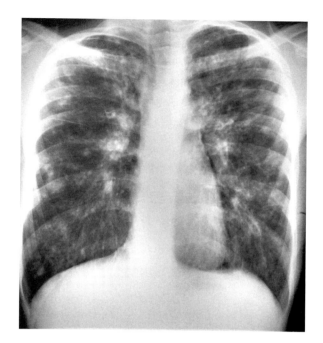

FIGURE 16-17

Posteroanterior chest radiograph shows predominantly upper lobe bronchiectasis, with multiple thick-walled, dilated, nontapering central airways. Note the large lung volumes as evidence of air-trapping and presumptive obliterative bronchiolitis.

Suggested Reading

Wood BP. Cystic fibrosis: 1997. *Radiology* 1997;204:1–10.

Congenital Bronchial Atresia

KEY FACTS

- Congenital bronchial atresia is a developmental anomaly caused by atresia of a segmental or lobar bronchus. The resulting blind-end bronchus has no connection to the rest of the tracheobronchial tree. Mucus secretion in the obstructed segment leads to a dilated, mucus-filled bronchus, a bronchocele.

- Bronchoceles can also be seen secondary to obstructing neoplasms of the bronchus such as carcinoid tumor and bronchogenic carcinoma and in nonobstructive disorders such as allergic bronchopulmonary aspergillosis, bronchocentric granulomatosis, and cystic fibrosis.

- The involved lung parenchyma is hyperinflated because of collateral ventilation through the pores of Kohn and canals of Lambert, allowing air to enter the involved lung segment, but without adequate exhalation.

- Patients usually present with an incidentally discovered, asymptomatic lung mass. On chest radiographs, the bronchocele is typically a smoothly marginated, perihilar structure often showing a branching V or Y-shaped configuration. The bronchocele is subtended by hyperinflated lung. Chest CT scanning better shows the characteristic branching pattern of a bronchocele over serial slices, and adjacent hyperinflated lung parenchyma.

- The most common sites of involvement include segmental bronchi in the left upper (apical-posterior), left lower, and right upper lobes.

- Patients typically require no treatment. Rarely, surgical intervention is warranted in the setting of recurrent lung infections or if ventilation of the adjacent lung is impaired from progressive hyperinflation.

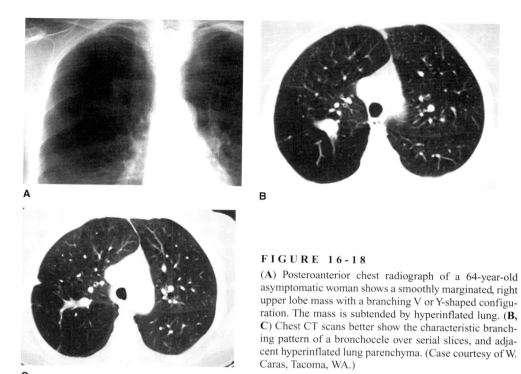

A

B

C

FIGURE 16-18

(**A**) Posteroanterior chest radiograph of a 64-year-old asymptomatic woman shows a smoothly marginated, right upper lobe mass with a branching V or Y-shaped configuration. The mass is subtended by hyperinflated lung. (**B, C**) Chest CT scans better show the characteristic branching pattern of a bronchocele over serial slices, and adjacent hyperinflated lung parenchyma. (Case courtesy of W. Caras, Tacoma, WA.)

Suggested Reading

Pugatch RD, Gale JE. Obscure pulmonary masses: bronchial impaction revealed by CT. *AJR* 1983;141:909–914.

17   Esophageal Diseases

Esophageal Carcinoma

KEY FACTS

- Esophageal carcinoma, the fifth most common malignancy, comprises about 10% of gastrointestinal tract tumors. Patients are usually aged more than 60 years and the 5-year survival is poor (< 10%).

- Most esophageal malignancies (90%) are squamous cell carcinomas that arise in the upper two thirds of the esophagus. The minority are adenocarcinomas related to columnar metaplasia in the distal one third of the esophagus, so-called "Barrett's esophagus," resulting from reflux esophagitis. Lymphoma is rare.

- Risk factors include cigarette smoking, excess alcohol consumption, lye stricture, achalasia, radiation therapy, and gastroesophageal reflux disease.

- On chest radiographs, proximal esophageal dilation caused by tumor is identified more readily than the tumor itself. Other radiographic signs include a mediastinal air–fluid level and fullness of the retrotracheal band and anterior displacement of the trachea on the lateral radiograph.

- Esophagram or endoscopy are used for screening. Esophagram shows mucosal destruction.

- Computed tomography (CT) scan shows surrounding tumor extent, local invasion into adjacent structures, and local metastases.

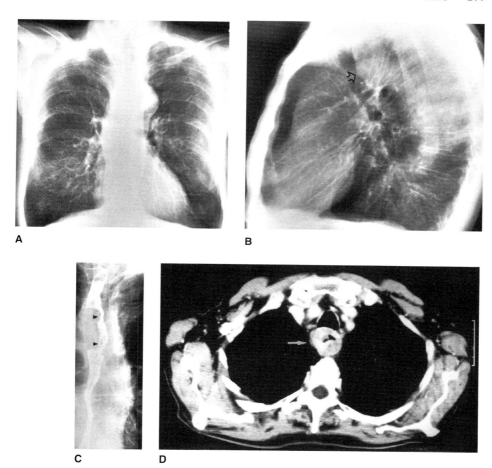

FIGURE 17-1 Frontal (**A**) and lateral (**B**) chest radiographs show slight widening of the superior mediastinum with a retrotracheal mass (*open arrow*). (**C**) Barium swallow shows narrowing of the midesophagus with destruction of mucosa (*arrowheads*). (**D**) CT scan shows marked thickening of the esophageal wall (*arrows*).

Suggested Reading

Putman CE, Curtis AM, Westfried M, et al. Thickening of the posterior tracheal stripe: a sign of squamous cell carcinoma of the esophagus. *Radiology* 1976;121:533–536.

Esophageal Leiomyoma

KEY FACTS

- Benign esophageal lesions are less common than esophageal malignancies.
- Esophageal leiomyoma comprises more than 50% of benign esophageal lesions.
- Esophageal leiomyoma is typically intramural and usually asymptomatic. Large tumors can cause dysphagia.
- Chest radiographs are usually normal but larger lesion may manifest as a middle mediastinal mass.
- Barium swallow shows an intramural lesion that may be calcified. Larger leiomyomas are visible on CT.
- Leiomyoma is not reliably distinguished from leiomyosarcoma on the basis of imaging features.

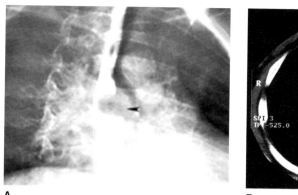
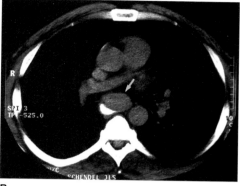

A   **B**

FIGURE 17-2   (**A**) Single image from a barium swallow shows mural filling defect (*arrowhead*) in the midesophagus. (**B**) CT scan shows a soft-tissue mass in the wall of the esophagus (*arrow*) that compresses the contrast-filled lumen. This proved to be an esophageal leiomyoma.

Suggested Reading

Plachta A. Benign tumors of the esophagus: review of the literature and report of 99 cases. *Am J Gastroenterol* 1962;38:639–652.

Achalasia

KEY FACTS

- Primary achalasia is caused be hypertonicity of the lower esophageal sphincter, leading to abnormal peristalsis.
- Secondary achalasia is caused by gastric carcinoma, lymphoma, or Chagas' disease.
- Patients with achalasia experience chest pain, dysphagia, and regurgitation.
- Chest radiographs show a very widened mediastinum, usually with a "double" right-side heart contour, convex to the right and often with air–fluid level on erect studies.
- Esophagography is diagnostic and shows esophageal dilation and a beaklike narrowing of the lower esophageal sphincter.
- Balloon dilation of the lower esophageal sphincter is the treatment of choice. Follow-up radiographs are necessary to observe for complications, namely an iatrogenic Boerhaave's syndrome (esophageal rupture).

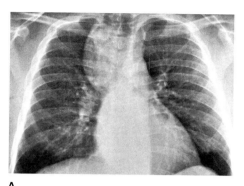

A

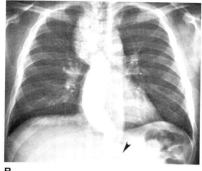

B

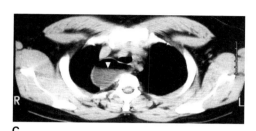

C

FIGURE 17-3

(**A**) Posteroanterior chest radiograph of a 35-year-old man shows widened right superior mediastinum. (**B**) Single image from a barium swallow shows a markedly dilated esophagus with beaklike tapering at the gastroesophageal junction (*arrowhead*). (**C**) On CT scan through the upper mediastinum, a markedly dilated esophagus is evident, which contains an air–fluid level (*arrowhead*).

Suggested Reading

Cole TJ, Turner MA. Manifestations of gastrointestinal disease on chest radiographs. *Radiographics* 1993;13:1013–1034.

Esophageal Rupture or Laceration

KEY FACTS

- Esophageal rupture can occur either from blunt (very rare) or penetrating injuries; it can also be a complication of instrumentation and vigorous emesis (Boerhaave's syndrome).

- Blunt injuries are usually seen in the phrenic ampulla and cervical esophagus, whereas penetrating injuries can occur anywhere, depending on the location of the entrance wound.

- Penetrating injuries that traverse the mediastinum require assessment of the great vessels (angiography), trachea (bronchoscopy), and esophagus (endoscopy and/or esophagography). Classically, each assessment misses one third of injuries, but not the same third.

- In penetrating injuries of the supraclavicular esophagus, the trachea is injured in one half the cases.

- Delay in diagnosing esophageal rupture doubles patient mortality every 6 hours; mortality is more than 85% if the delay is more than 24 hours.

- Chest radiographs are nonspecific, usually showing a wide mediastinum and left pleural effusion or hydropneumothorax. Pneumomediastinum is another common, nonspecific finding. Occasionally, the V-sign of Naclerio is seen where the pneumomediastinum extends to and reflects the parietal pleura off the left hemidiaphragm, yielding a lucent "V" shape.

- Pleural effusion often shows low pH and high amylase levels.

- Mediastinitis and abscess formation can result from an esophageal laceration.

- For esophagographic diagnosis of esophageal rupture, use nonionic contrast (300 mg I/mL) in the left anterior oblique (LAO) position. If this is normal, follow with thin barium solution in the LAO and right anterior oblique (RAO) positions.

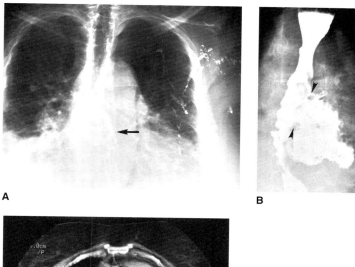

A

B

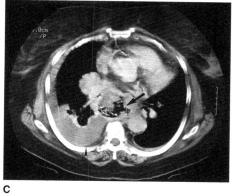

C

FIGURE 17-4

(**A**) Frontal chest radiograph shows extra-luminal contrast in the mediastinum (*arrow*). (**B**) Barium swallow shows a broad-based site of rupture (*arrowheads*). (**C**) CT scan shows extraluminal air in the mediastinum (*arrow*) and a left pleural effusion (*arrowhead*). A ruptured esophageal cancer was discovered at surgery.

Suggested Reading

Bjerke HS. Penetrating and blunt injuries of the esophagus. *Chest Surg Clin North Am* 1994; 4:811–818.

Paraesophageal Varices

KEY FACTS

- Paraesophageal varices are collateral vessels that form in response to portal venous hypertension, usually in the setting of hepatic cirrhosis.
- Upper gastrointestinal bleeding is more common from paraesophageal varices than from other portosystemic collateral vessels.
- On chest radiographs, paraesophageal varices may appear as retrocardiac density with a smooth or lobulated contour. They can cause loss of the descending aorta silhouette. Often they are not seen at all.
- On barium study, serpiginous filling defect are identified in the lower esophagus.
- On CT, serpiginous densities are seen adjacent to or within the distal esophagus and enhance with intravenous contrast media.
- After sclerotherapy, pleural effusions and added mediastinal opacity may be evident.

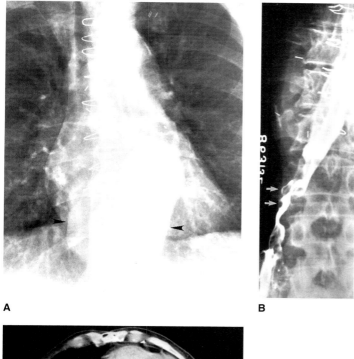

A   B

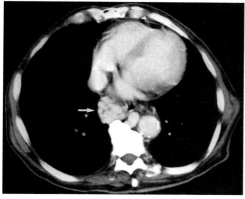

C

FIGURE 17-5

(**A**) Posteroanterior chest radiograph of a man with cirrhosis shows bilateral abnormal inferior mediastinal interfaces (*arrowheads*). (**B**) Esophagram shows narrowing of the distal esophagus with serpiginous filling defects (*arrows*). (**C**) CT scan through the inferior mediastinum shows enhancing tubular structures (*arrow*), which represent paraesophageal varices.

Suggested Reading

Ishikawa T, Saeki M, Tsukune Y, et al. Detection of paraesophageal varices by plain films. *AJR* 1985;144:701–704.

Esophageal Duplication Cyst

KEY FACTS

- Esophageal duplication cysts are foregut lesions such as bronchogenic cysts, but instead they arise from abnormal differentiation of the posterior bud of the developing tracheobronchial tree.
- The cyst wall contains gastrointestinal tract epithelium.
- Most cysts are located adjacent to the esophagus.
- Cysts are usually asymptomatic but can cause dysphagia if they are large.
- Cysts can contain air if they communicate with the tracheobronchial tree. In such cases, the possibility of infection should be considered, which usually necessitates surgical removal.
- Barium swallow shows an extrinsic lesion. CT scan show a well-marginated lesion adjacent to the esophagus with contents of fluid density. Distinguishing between esophageal duplication cyst and bronchogenic cyst can be difficult.

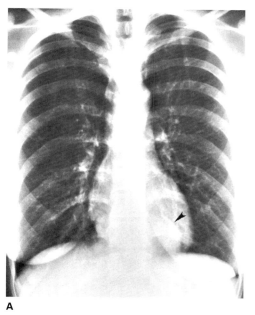

A

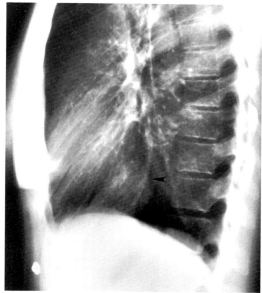

B

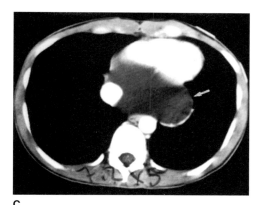

C

FIGURE 17-6

Posteroanterior (**A**) and lateral (**B**) chest radiographs show a soft tissue density (*arrowheads*) posterior to the heart. (**C**) CT scan shows a fluid density cyst (*arrow*) posterior to the contrast-enhanced heart.

Suggested Reading

Fitch SJ, Tonkin ILD, Tonkin AK. Imaging of foregut duplication cysts. *Radiographics* 1986; 6:189–201.

Esophageal Candidiasis (AIDS)

KEY FACTS

- Esophageal candidiasis is an early and frequent manifestation in patients with acquired immune deficiency syndrome (AIDS).
- Dysphagia is the most common presenting symptom.
- Barium esophagram is most suggestive and early in the disease course shows edematous folds.
- In later stages, candidiasis produces widespread plaque formation and multiple deep ulcers.
- Large discrete ulcers are more typical of cytomegalovirus than of candidiasis.
- Computed tomography scans may show diffuse esophageal thickening but otherwise is nonspecific.

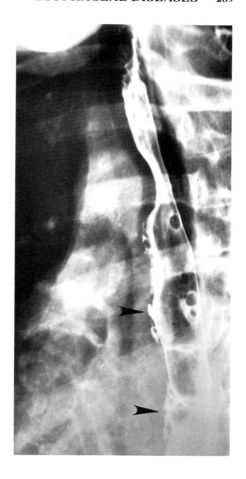

FIGURE 17-7

Single image from a barium swallow in a human immun-odeficiency (HIV)-positive patient shows multiple small ulcerations in the esophageal wall (*arrowheads*) caused by candidiasis. (Courtesy of Thorsten Krebs, MD.)

Suggested Reading

Frager DH, Frager JD, Brandt LJ, et al. Gastrointestinal complications of AIDS: radiological feature. *Radiology* 1986;158:597–603.

Hiatal Hernia

KEY FACTS

- Hiatal hernia is a gastric herniation that occurs through the esophageal hiatus. Usually, the gastric fundus is affected.
- Hiatal hernia is very common, and it is reported in more than half of elderly patients.
- Two types of hiatal hernias are recognized. A sliding hiatal hernia occurs if the gastroesophageal junction is displaced upward into the mediastinum. Sliding hiatal hernias are often small and reducible. A paraesophageal hernia, which is less common, is characterized by normal location of the gastroesophageal junction and herniation of a part of the fundus through the diaphragm adjacent to the gastroesophageal junction.
- A paraesophageal hernia may not reduce and it can be complicated by incarceration or volvulus. Surgical repair may be necessary.
- The chest radiograph of hiatal hernia shows a retrocardiac density that may contain an air–fluid level.
- The diagnosis can be confirmed on barium swallow or cross-sectional imaging.

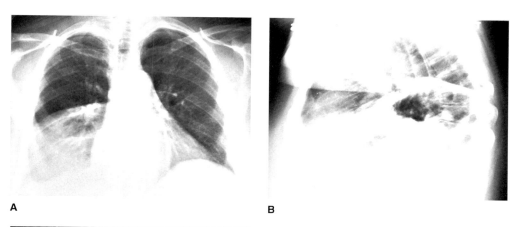

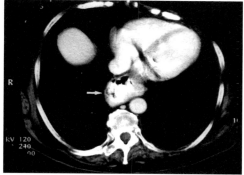

FIGURE 17-8

Posteroanterior (**A**) and lateral (**B**) chest radiographs show a large air-filled soft-tissue density in the lower chest caused by a hiatal hernia. (**C**) CT scan through the lower chest in a different patient shows contrast and air in a hiatal hernia (*arrowhead*).

Suggested Reading

Levine MS. Gastroesophageal junction. In: Levine MS, ed. *Radiology of the esophagus.* Philadelphia: WB Saunders, 1989:247–265.

Esophageal Diverticula

- Esophageal diverticula are outpouchings of the esophagus. True diverticula contain all layers of the esophagus.
- Pulsion diverticula commonly affect the lower esophagus, and they are caused by excessive intraluminal pressure.
- Traction diverticula, which typically affect the midesophagus, are caused by retraction by an adjacent inflammatory disease such as tuberculous lymphadenopathy.
- Zencker's diverticulum occurs in an area of potential muscular weakness called "Killian's dehiscence" just above the cricopharyngeal sphincter.
- Zencker's diverticula are thus located in the hypopharynx. They most often project posteriorly and leftward.
- On contrast studies, diverticula are recognized as outpouchings of the esophagus or hypopharynx.

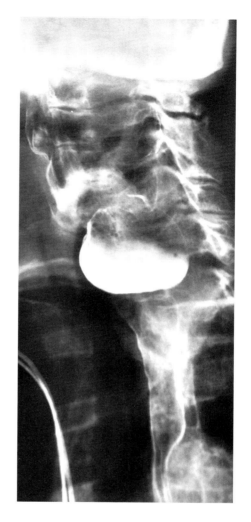

FIGURE 17-9
Single view from a barium swallow shows a pocket of retained contrast medium extending from the hypopharynx, which represents a Zenker's diverticulum.

Suggested Reading

Reddy ER, Smith I, Clarke H. Esophageal diverticula. *Can Assoc Radiol J* 1989;40:306.

18 Great Vessel Abnormalities

Atherosclerosis

KEY FACTS

- Atherosclerosis is a subtype of arteriosclerosis that involves the formation of patchy, nodular plaques in the larger arteries including the aorta, coronary artery, and the aortic arch vessels. Among men and women, it is the leading cause of death in the United States; it leads to ischemic heart disease and stroke.

- Certain disease processes are associated with premature atherosclerosis: diabetes mellitus, hypertension, hypercholesterolemia, combined hyperlipidemia, hypothyroidism, and systemic lupus erythematosis, among others. Other factors that play a role in athersclerotic plaque formation include cigarette smoking, obesity, physical inactivity, stress, male gender, and genetic factors.

- The normal, diffuse, progressive, age-related thickening of the vascular intima should be distinguished from the focal, discrete, raised plaques of atherosclerosis.

- Angiography is the best test for showing a focal plaque within the lumen of a vessel. This does not necessarily imply any clinical or physiologic significance. Radiographic demonstration of calcification within a vessel wall strongly implies atherosclerosis, but does not demonstrate all atherosclerotic plaques, as not all plaques are calcified.

- Spiral computed tomography (CT) angiography can potentially evaluate the thoracic aorta and its branches for aortic aneurysm, aortic dissection, Takayasu arteritis, and penetrating aortic atherosclerotic ulcer. Advantages of CT angiography include thin axial sections showing mural changes, high contrast resolution and high sensitivity for detecting calcified lesions, and angiographic or three-dimensional display of vascular structures and adjacent organs in any projection with a single spiral acquisition.

- Intravascular ultrasound, transesophageal echocardiography, and magnetic resonance imaging (MRI) are some potential imaging tools under investigation for the assessment of atherosclerosis. With current cine techniques and three-dimensional MRI angiography, the thoracic aorta can be examined noninvasively with a high degree of accuracy.

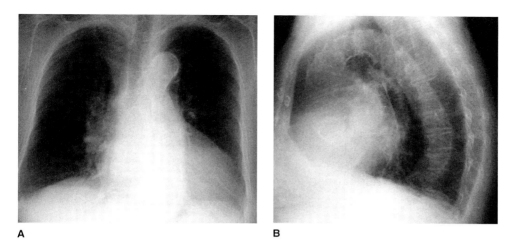

A   **B**

F I G U R E   1 8 - 1   Posteroanterior **(A)** and lateral **(B)** chest radiographs of a 84-year-old man show dense calcification of the wall of the entire thoracic aorta. Although somewhat tortuous, the aorta is nondilated. This is a typical appearance of the senescent, usually atherosclerotic aorta. Also seen is associated cardiomegaly, but no evidence of left heart failure.

Suggested Reading

Chung JW, Park JH, Im JG, et al. Spiral CT angiography of the thoracic aorta. *Radiographics* 1996;16:811–824.

Coronary Artery Calcification

KEY FACTS

- With the advent of improved contrast resolution and rapid CT scan times, visualization of coronary artery calcifications is now commonplace.
- Calcification within coronary arteries usually signifies atherosclerosis. The incidence of coronary artery calcification increases with patient age, paralleling the increased incidence of coronary atherosclerosis with advancing age.
- Region of interest (ROI) measurements permit an objective measurement of tissue density, but qualitative imaging will usually suffice.
- In an asymptomatic younger patient, coronary artery calcifications may represent nonflow limiting plaque—plaque that can rupture and lead to sudden death.
- The early detection of coronary artery calcifications can lead to preventative lifestyle changes. The efficacy of screening programs has yet to be determined.

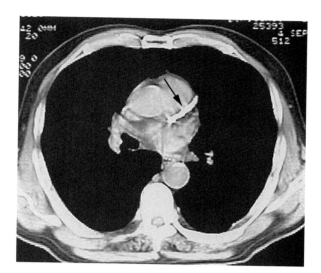

FIGURE 18-2

Computed tomography scan through the aortic root of a 66-year-old man shows extensive arterial calcification of the left anterior descending coronary artery (*arrow*).

Suggested Reading

Rumberger JA, Sheedy PF 2nd, Breen JF, et al. Electron beam CT and coronary artery disease: scanning for coronary artery calcification *Mayo Clin Proc* 1996;71:369–377.

Aortic Aneurysm

KEY FACTS

- An aortic aneurysm is a localized or diffuse aortic dilation caused by weakness or a structural defect within the aortic wall that can present in a wide variety of shapes, sizes, and locations.
- Approximately one fourth of all arteriosclerotic aneurysms involve the thoracic aorta.
- Aneurysms of the thoracic aorta can be classified anatomically into five groups based on location: (a) ascending aorta; (b) transverse aortic arch; (c) distal to left subclavian artery; (d) descending thoracic aorta; and (e) thoracoabdominal aorta.
- True aneurysms have all layers of the vessel wall intact. False aneurysms have none of the layers intact. Pseudoaneurysms have one or two of the layers of the vessel wall intact.
- Saccular aneurysms involve only a focal portion of the vessel wall, whereas fusiform aneurysms involve the vessel wall circumferentially. Most thoracic aneurysms are fusiform but up to 20% are saccular.
- The most common cause for thoracic aortic aneurysms is arteriosclerosis. Other causes include connective tissue diseases, trauma, neoplastic invasion, and infection. Syphilitic aneurysms and mycotic aneurysms are often saccular; although, syphilitic aneurysms occur most commonly in the ascending aorta.
- With the saccular type aneurysms, chest radiographs often show a nonspecific rounded opacity contiguous with the thoracic aorta. The differential diagnosis includes benign or malignant lung neoplasms as well as a mediastinal mass. A vascular cause for this radiographic appearance should always be considered in the differential diagnosis; biopsies should not be performed until an aneurysm has been excluded.
- Spiral CT and MRI reliably evaluate the size, location, and extent of aneurysmal disease. Contrast CT scanning shows marked luminal enhancement. The periphery of the aneurysm may contain thrombus.
- Aneurysms are often found incidentally. Chest pain and symptoms related to compression of adjacent structures occur. If sufficiently large, the aneurysm(s) can compress the left main or lower lobe bronchus with associated atelectasis. Dysphagia can occur if the esophagus is compressed. Enlarging aneurysms and those greater than 6 cm are at risk for rupture, which usually is fatal.
- Do not confuse aortic aneurysms with aortic dissection.

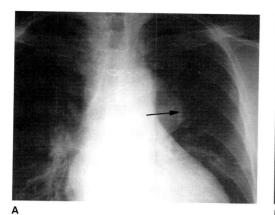 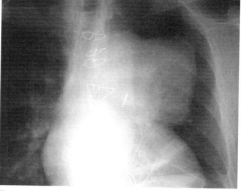

A   **B**

FIGURE 18-3   (A) Posteroanterior chest radiograph of a 70-year-old man with vague chest pain shows a moderate-sized focal aneurysm of the descending thoracic aorta (*arrow*). (B) Eight years later, the aneurysm, left untreated, has markedly increased in size.

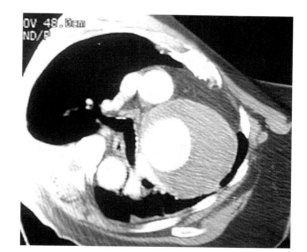

FIGURE 18-4

Computed tomography scan through the aortic arch of a 75-year-old man shows a 13 cm focal aneurysm of the descending thoracic aorta arising near the ductus diverticulum. Note the large amount of thrombus within the aneurysm.

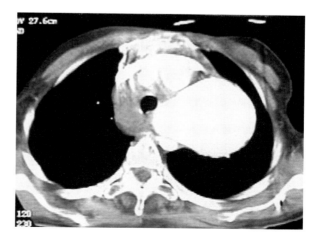

FIGURE 18-5

Computed tomography scan through the aortic arch of a 77-year-old man shows a large contrast-filled saccular aneurysm of the aortic arch. In this case, no thrombus is seen within the aneurysm.

Suggested Reading

Posniak HV, Olson MC, Demos TC, et al. CT of thoracic aortic aneurysms. *Radiographics* 1990;10:839–855.

Aortic Dissection

KEY FACTS

- Acute thoracic aortic dissection (AAD) is the most common emergency affecting the aorta; its incidence exceeds that of ruptures of thoracic and abdominal aneurysm combined. Untreated, AAD can be rapidly fatal; 36% to 72% of patients die within 48 hours and 62% to 91% within the first week.

- Advances in surgical repair and antihypertensive medication, have markedly improved survival.

- Noninvasive imaging provides prompt and reliable diagnosis of AAD; it has largely supplanted aortography, which will not be discussed.

- The original DeBakey classification of AAD has been replaced by the Stanford classification, which divides AAD into surgical and nonsurgical groups. Dissection involving any portion of the aorta proximal to the origin of the left subclavian artery (Stanford type A) usually requires emergency surgical repair, whereas dissection confined to the descending aorta (Stanford type B) usually requires only management of hypertension.

- Patients with hypertension or with connective tissue disorders such as Marfan's syndrome, cystic medial necrosis, and Ehlers-Danlos and Turner's syndromes are at risk for AAD. Pregnancy, aortic stenosis, and coarctation of the aorta are other risk factors.

- Chest radiographic findings supportive of AAD include progressive aortic enlargement on serial examinations, double contour of the aortic arch, and more than 6 mm displacement of intimal calcification. Apparent displacement of intimal calcification can be a projectional artifact when calcification in the anterior part of the aortic arch is projected over the descending aorta. In the absence of comparison radiographs showing acute enlargement, an enlarged arch is not specific for the diagnosis; it is usually the result of hypertension or atherosclerosis.

- Furthermore, a normal configuration of the arch should not be interpreted as excluding AAD, because the arch may appear normal in 25% of cases of AAD. Other radiographic findings supporting the diagnosis of AAD include a new pleural effusion and pericardial effusion.

- Classic findings of AAD on CT are an intimal flap and false lumen, as found in approximately 70% of cases; demonstration of the intimal flap is usually conclusive. Secondary findings include increased attenuation of the acutely thrombosed false lumen on precontrast scans, internal displacement of intimal calcifications, mediastinal or pericardial hematoma, delayed opacification of the false lumen, mural thickening with increased attenuation, and irregular compression of the true lumen by expanding intramural hematoma or thrombus. Ischemia or infarction of organs supplied by branch vessels from the false lumen is an important secondary finding.

- As MRI evolves, its accuracy continues to increase. Recent diagnostic sensitivity and specificity have been reported to be 98.3% and 97.8%, respectively, although other reports indicate considerable dependence on the experience of the observer. As on CT scans, the classic finding of AAD with MRI is an intimal flap, the signal within the false lumen is variable, depending on the blood flow, the presence, age, and composition of thrombus, and the pulse sequence. Intimal calcification is usually not visible with MRI. Spin-echo MRI typically shows flow voids within both the false and true lumens. The intimal flap is then visible as an intervening stripe of soft-tissue signal. Flow-related signal changes may demonstrate aortic insufficiency or differences in flow between adjacent channels.

- As with CT, findings supporting the diagnosis of AAD include pericardial or pleural effusion, mediastinal hemorrhage, and aortic wall thickening. MRI can be difficult to perform in the acutely ill patient because of the relatively long examination time, the susceptibility to motion artifacts, the need for regular cardiac rhythm, and difficulties in patient monitoring.

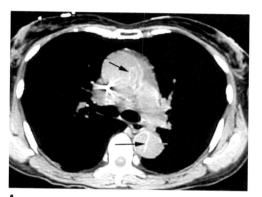

A

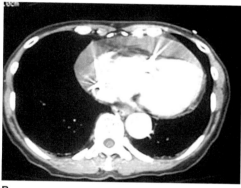

B

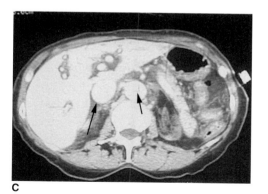

C

FIGURE 18-6

Pre- and postcontrast CT scan of the chest and abdomen of a 70-year-old woman with cardiac tamponade physiology shows the displaced intimal flaps on the noncontrast scan (*arrows*) **(A)** and a pericardial fluid collection **(B)**. **(C)** Note the aortic dissection (*short arrow*), the distended inferior vena cava (*long arrow*), and the periportal edema, which was caused by the cardiac tamponade.

Suggested Reading

Rubin GD. Helical CT angiography of the thoracic aorta. *J Thorac Imaging* 1997;12:128–149.

Acute Traumatic Aortic Injury

KEY FACTS

- Traumatic injury to the thoracic aorta accounts for 15% to 20% of fatalities in high-speed deceleration accidents; 85% to 90% of these victims die at the accident scene.

- Of the 10% to 15% of patients who reach the hospital; 30% die within 6 hours, 40% to 50% die within 24 hours, and 90% die within 4 months if the aortic injury is not discovered and repaired.

- Traumatic thoracic aortic injuries occur most commonly at the aortic isthmus (80% to 85%), followed by the ascending aortic arch (5% to 9%), aortic branches (4% to 10%), and diaphragmatic hiatus (1% to 3%).

- Chronic post-traumatic thoracic aortic pseudoaneurysm develops in 2% to 5% of patients with this injury. Only rarely do these patients live a normal life span.

- Many chest radiographic signs are used to detect mediastinal hematoma; therefore, none of these signs are very sensitive or specific for acute traumatic aortic injury. The mechanism of injury and clinical suspicion are still important factors. The best and most reliable chest radiographic signs of mediastinal hematoma and, thus, indirectly of acute traumatic aortic injury include:

     Superior mediastinal widening (>8 cm)

     Loss of the normally sharp aortic contour or a double contour to the arch

     Nasogastric tube deviation to the right

     Tracheal deviation

     Left apical capping

     Depression of left main bronchus

- Mediastinal widening on the chest radiograph is the most sensitive diagnostic sign for traumatic aortic injury (> 90%); however, by itself, it is not that useful, with a specificity of only 10%.

- A normal aortic contour, aorticopulmonary window, left paraspinal and right paratracheal interface, and absence of deviation of the nasogastric tube has a greater than 98% probability of no aortic rupture.

- Differential diagnosis for mediastinal widening includes mediastinal lipomatosis, sternal dislocation, and thoracic spine fracture with paraspinous hematoma.

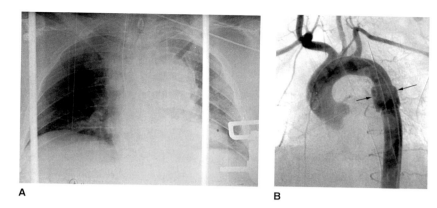

A   **B**

FIGURE 18-7   (**A**) Anteroposterior chest radiograph of a 52-year-old-man hit by a car shows superior mediastinal widening, deviation of the nasogastric and endotracheal tubes to the right, and loss of the normally sharp aortic contour. These findings, as well as the mechanism of injury indicated aortography. (**B**) Left anterior oblique aortic angiogram shows a typical aortic laceration at the aortic isthmus (*arrows*).

Suggested Reading

Woodring JH, Loh FK, Kryscio RJ. Mediastinal hemorrhage: an evaluation of radiographic manifestations. *Radiology* 1984;151:15–21.

Chronic Aortic Pseudoaneurysm

KEY FACTS

- Traumatic aortic injury is most often caused by a high-speed motor vehicle accident.
- Nearly all surviving patients have injuries in the proximal descending aorta just distal to the left subclavian artery.
- If unrecognized, most patients with an untreated aortic laceration will die, but occasionally, the laceration will evolve into a chronic aortic pseudoaneurysm. The patient may present incidentally with radiographic evidence of a chronic aortic pseudoaneurysm many years after the injury.
- Radiographically, the chronic pseudoaneurysm manifests as an outpouching of the proximal descending aorta. Rim calcification is frequently present.
- Computed tomography and MRI scans show the lesion more clearly and can define the neck of the pseudoaneurysm.
- Chronic aortic pseudoaneurysms can rupture; when discovered, surgical resection is usually recommended.

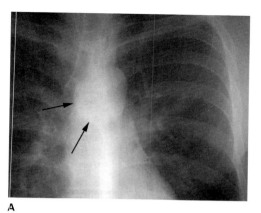

A

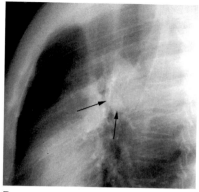

B

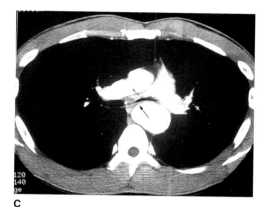

C

FIGURE 18-8

Posteroanterior (**A**) and lateral (**B**) chest radiograph of a 32-year-old-man who was involved in a motorcycle accident 9 years earlier presented with this abnormal aortic contour. Note the mass in the middle mediastinum abutting the aortic arch (*arrows*). (**C**) CT scan through the mass shows a focal aneurysmal dilation of the aorta at the level of the ligamentum arteriosum (*arrow*), in this case, caused by a rare chronic pseudoaneurysm that had gone undetected.

Suggested Reading

Stark P. Traumatic rupture of the thoracic aorta: a review. *Crit Rev Diagn Imaging* 1986;21: 229–255.

Aberrant Subclavian Artery

KEY FACTS

- Aberrant right subclavian artery (ARSA) is a common arch anomaly that occurs in 0.5% of individuals. Rarely, an aberrant left subclavian artery can arise from a right-sided aortic arch.
- The aberrant vessel arises as the most distal branch of the aortic arch and courses rightward, posterior to the esophagus, prior to assuming its normal position in the right superior mediastinum.
- The ARSA is usually an incidental finding. However, a small proportion of patients have difficulty caused by posterior indentation of the esophagus, a symptom called "dysphagia lusoria."
- The origin of the aberrant vessel may be enlarged, causing a diverticulum of Kommerel. The vessel occasionally is aneurysmal.
- The frontal chest radiograph is frequently normal, but can show an oblique interface in the mediastinum extending rightward and cephalad because of the anomalous vessel. Anterior bowing of the trachea may be found on the lateral radiograph.
- A characteristic posterior indentation is present on the upper part of a contrast-filled esophagus.
- Both CT and MRI scanning best show the typical retroesophageal course of the aberrant vessel and any dilation.

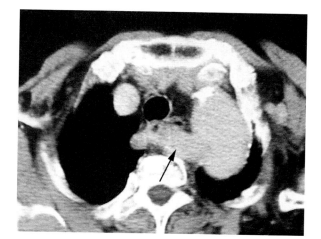

FIGURE 18-9

Computed tomography scan of a 76-year-old man shows a tubular mass arising from the aorta and coursing behind the trachea and esophagus (*arrow*), typical for an aberrant right subclavian artery.

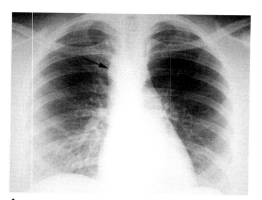

A

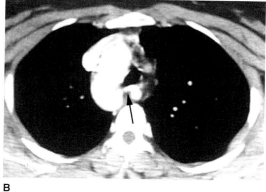

B

FIGURE 18-10   (**A**) Posteroanterior chest radiograph shows an incidental right aortic arch (*arrow*). (**B**) Contrast-enhanced CT scan through the level of the aortic arch shows an enhancing aortic branch artery coursing behind the trachea and esophagus (*arrow*), typical for an aberrant left subclavian artery.

Suggested Reading

Proto AV, Cuthbert NW, Raider L. Aberrant right subclavian artery: further observations. *AJR* 1987;148:253–257.

Persistent Left Superior Vena Cava

KEY FACTS

- A persistent left superior vena cava is a normal variant that occurs in 0.3% of otherwise healthy individuals. It is seen in 4.3% of patients with congenital heart disease.

- Persistent left superior vena cava is caused embryologically by lack of involution of the left anterior and common cardinal veins.

- The right superior vena cava is typically smaller than normal or is absent.

- In 40% of cases, the left brachiocephalic vein connecting the right and left cavae is absent.

- The left superior vena cava provides drainage for the left internal jugular and left subclavian veins.

- The persistent vessel courses inferiorly through the left mediastinum to terminate in the coronary sinus. In patients with congenital heart disease, the left superior vena cava may drain directly into the left atrium.

- The frontal radiograph may show widening of the left superior mediastinum, but the usual recognition is from an apparently misplaced central venous catheter into a normal left superior vena cava.

- Computed tomography and MRI scanning best show the course of the normal variant vessel and any associated anomalies.

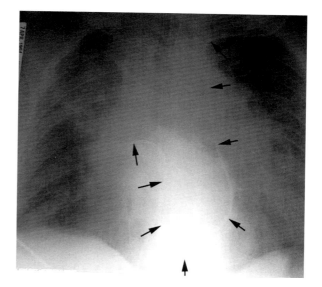

FIGURE 18-11
Anteroposterior chest radiograph of a 45-year-old man with a pulmonary artery catheter in an unusual location; within a normal persistent left superior vena cava (*arrows* show course of the catheter).

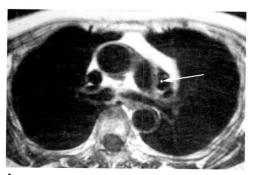

A

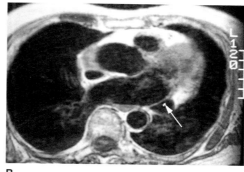

B

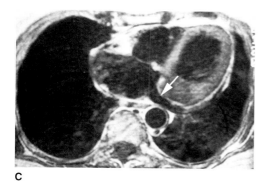

C

FIGURE 18-12
Serial axial MRI scans show a normal persistent left superior vena cava (PLSVC) (*arrows*). **(A)** At the level of the carina, the PLSVC is lateral to the aorta and main pulmonary artery. **(B)** At the level of the left atrium, the PLSVC sweeps behind the left atrium. **(C)** At the level of the right atrium, the PLSVC drains into the coronary sinus and right atrium, as expected.

Suggested Reading

White CS, Baffa JM, Haney PJ, et al. MR imaging of congenital anomalies of the thoracic veins. *Radiographics* 1997;17:595–608.

Congenital Interruption of the Inferior Vena Cava with Azygous Continuation

KEY FACTS

- The incidence of congenital interruption of the inferior vena cava (IVC) with continuation through the azygous venous system has been reported to range from less than 1% to 2%.

- Most cases are asymptomatic and may be discovered incidentally on routine chest radiographs. They are usually detected on frontal radiographs as an "end on," round, or oval shadow at right tracheobronchial angle.

- Causes of azygous vein dilation include, most commonly, elevated central venous pressure (e.g., cardiac decompensation, pericardial diseases such as acute pericardial tamponade or constrictive pericarditis, or tricuspid valve diseases). Other causes include obstruction of either the superior or inferior vena cava, portal hypertension, hepatic vein obstruction, anomalous pulmonary venous drainage, and congenital azygous continuation of an interrupted IVC, where it reaches its largest size.

- When the diagnosis is suggested, a chest CT scan is helpful in showing the anatomy. MRI is also helpful for detailed study of other associated anomalies such as the cardiosplenic syndromes.

- The embryogenesis of the IVC is controversial. Generally it is formed by the development, regression, and anastomosis of three pairs of primitive channels: the posterior cardinal, subcardinal, and supracardinal veins. The failure of the union between the hepatic and the right subcardinal veins and the persistence, instead of regression, of the supracardinal veins result in the absence of the infrahepatic IVC with azygous or hemiazygous continuation, respectively.

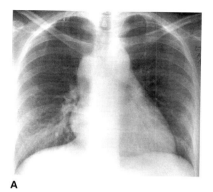

A

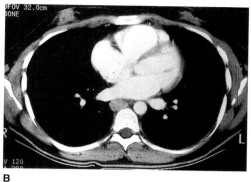

B

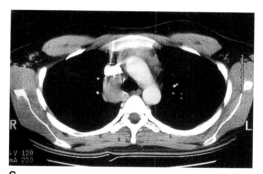

C

FIGURE 18-13

(**A**) Posteroanterior chest radiograph of a 22-year-old man who sustained minor trauma after a bicycle accident shows a rounded opacity in the right tracheobronchial angle. (**B**) CT scan of the chest at the level of the left atrium shows a large azygous vein that extends all the way down in the abdomen. An inferior vena cava would have emptied in the right atrium at this level. (**C**) Chest CT scan showing the dilated azygous vein arching over the right main bronchus and draining in the superior vena cava.

Suggested Reading

Gharib AM, Stern EJ. Azygous vein enlargement mimicking adenopathy. *Clinical Pulmonary Medicine* 1997;4:355–356.

Azygous Fissure and Lobe

KEY FACTS

- The azygous fissure is an incidental finding of a normal variant that occurs in 0.4% of a individuals. It is formed embryologically by traversal of the azygos vein into the right upper lobe.
- The fissure consists of four pleural layers: two visceral and two parietal.
- The medial portion of the right upper lobe demarcated by the azygos fissure is sometimes called the "azygos lobe." However, no separate lobar bronchial supply is present. Bronchial supply is most often from the apical segmental bronchus.
- The fissure is identified on frontal radiographs as an oblique curvilinear structure that extends obliquely across the right upper lobe a variable distance from the mediastinum.
- At its inferior extent, the shadow widens into a teardrop-shaped form that corresponds to the azygous vein arch. No vein is present in the normal location at the right tracheobronchial angle.
- On CT scanning, the azygos arch is more cephalic than normal and lung protrudes posterior to the superior vena cava.
- The "azygos lobe" can be involved by pneumonia or cancer.

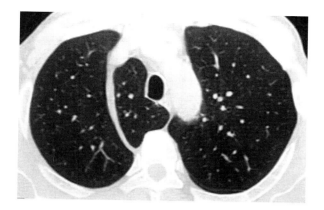

FIGURE 18-14
Computed tomography scan through the upper chest shows a tubular opacity representing the normal azygous vein, within an azygous fissure, creating the azygous lobe.

Suggested Reading

Felson B. The lobes and interlobar pleura: fundamental roentgen considerations. *Am J Med Sci* 1955;230:572.

Pulmonary Arterial Hypertension

KEY FACTS

- Pulmonary arterial hypertension (PAH) is caused by increased pulmonary vascular resistance or excessive pulmonary arterial flow.
- Specific causes of PAH can be classified as precapillary, pulmonary parenchymal, or postcapillary.
- Precapillary causes of PAH arise from the pulmonary arteries and include Eisenmenger's phenomenon, thromboembolic disease, and primary pulmonary hypertension.
- Pulmonary parenchymal causes of PAH include pulmonary emphysema and chronic interstitial lung disease. In these cases, increased pulmonary vascular resistance is caused by local hypoxia and vaso-obliteration.
- Postcapillary causes of PAH include congestive left heart failure, particularly that caused by mitral stenosis; pulmonary venous stenosis; and pulmonary veno-occlusive disease.
- The radiographic appearance of PAH depends on the specific cause. Precapillary PAH manifests as enlarged central pulmonary arteries with distal tapering or pruning. The right ventricle is enlarged on the lateral radiograph. In pulmonary parenchymal PAH, the enlarged central pulmonary arteries are accompanied by substantial abnormalities of the lung parenchyma. Postcapillary PAH shows a combination of enlarged central pulmonary arteries and changes of pulmonary venous hypertension.
- On CT scan, a mosaic pattern of lung attenuation can be present in the lung parenchyma; it can consist of alternating areas of hyper and hypoperfusion.

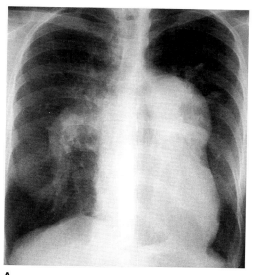

A

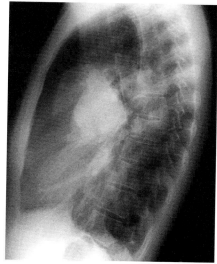

B

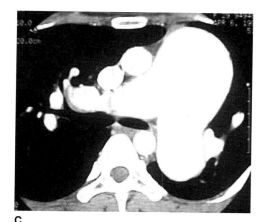

C

FIGURE 18-15

Posteroanterior (**A**) and lateral (**B**) chest radiographs of a 29-year-old woman show massive dilation of the central pulmonary arteries, in this case caused by an unrepaired atrial septal defect. Note the association pruning of the peripheral vascular markings. (**C**) Corresponding contrast-enhanced CT scan through the main pulmonary artery again shows massive dilation of the central arteries with a rapid decrease in vessel caliber that is typical of central pruning.

Suggested Reading

Simon M. Radiology of pulmonary hemodynamic disturbances and thromboembolism. In: Taveras JM, Ferrucci JT, eds. *Radiology: diagnosis-imaging-intervention*. Philadelphia: JB Lippincott, 1986;71:1–15.

Aortitis

KEY FACTS

- The differential diagnosis of aortitis includes inflammatory arthropathies (rheumatoid arthritis and Reiter's disease), granulomatous vasculitis, infection (syphilis and tuberculosis), radiation vasculitis, and rheumatic fever.

- Takayasu arteritis is a rare idiopathic, systemic, granulomatous vasculitis, also known as "pulseless disease," in reference to the peripheral pulse deficits that may develop. The pathologic lesions are similar to temporal arteritis, as both are giant cell arteritides, but the anatomic distribution of disease differs; Takayasu arteritis primarily affects the aorta and its major branches and rarely extends beyond the carotid bifurcation. Temporal arteritis does not involve the aorta.

- This disease process is most common in young females of reproductive years, (female to male ratio is 9:1), and it is more common in those of Asian descent.

- Two stages of the disease have been described. The acute stage is marked by nonspecific symptoms such as fever, myalgia, arthralgia, and malaise. The fibrotic stage is manifest as pulse deficits, claudication, bruits, and renovascular hypertension.

- Chest radiographic findings are minimal and nonspecific. Aortic obstruction can result in inferior rib notching secondary to collateral flow through the intercostal arteries. Calcification of the aortic wall can occur.

- Computed tomography scanning shows marked circumferential inflammatory thickening of the walls of the aorta and great vessels, which is a manifestation of granulomatous vasculitis.

- Arteriography shows long or short segments of smooth narrowing or stenoses of the proximal branches of the aorta along with focal narrowing of the thoracic and abdominal aorta. Associated aneurysms are seen in up to 25% of these patients.

- Treatment for this entity is often repeated and long-term immunosuppressive therapy (glucocorticoids alone or with a cytotoxic agent). Angioplasty, endovascular stent placement, and surgical bypass are also used in therapy.

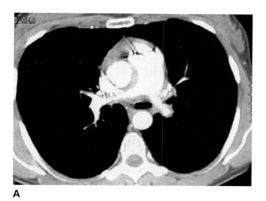 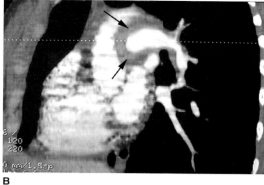

A **B**

FIGURE 18-16   Contrast-enhanced CT scan **(A)** at the level of the main pulmonary artery and an oblique reformation of a 13-year-old girl with Takayasu's arteritis **(B)** shows marked circumferential thickening of the pulmonary arteries (*arrows*) and aorta.

Suggested Reading

Cid MC, Font C, Coll-Vinent B, et al. Large vessel vasculitides. *Curr Opin Rheumatol* 1998; 10:18–28.

19 Heart and Pericardial Diseases

Chronic Congestive Heart Failure

KEY FACTS

- Chronic congestive heart failure (CHF) usually is caused by a decrease in systolic function. However, abnormal diastolic function and high output states can also cause CHF.

- Ischemia is an important cause of CHF. Other causes include valvular heart disease, cardiomyopathy (collagen vascular, drug toxicity, nutritional), and inflammatory (viral) myocarditis.

- High output forms of CHF are caused by chronic anemia, thyrotoxicosis, and pregnancy.

- The radiographic appearance of chronic CHF is dependent on its cause. The heart is typically enlarged, either globally or with a left ventricular configuration. Pericardial effusion can have a very similar appearance. Radiographic features reflect changes caused by heart chamber dilation. Hypertrophy may not change radiographic appearance; hypertrophy occurs at the expense of cavity volume.

- Calcification caused by a previous infarction or aneurysm can occur in the left ventricular wall.

- Pulmonary venous hypertension findings can be present. These include cephalization (redistribution) of pulmonary venous flow, interstitial (Kerley's) lines, and parenchymal edema.

- In advanced cases, pulmonary hemosiderosis characterized by chronic reticulonodular shadows in the lungs can occur. With nodular calcification of the hemosiderin deposits present, the term "pulmonary ossification" is used.

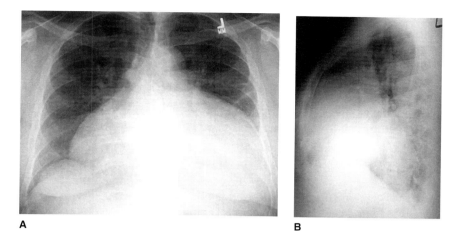

A   **B**

FIGURE 19-1   Posteroanterior (**A**) and lateral (**B**) chest radiographs of a 52-year-old man with a known ischemic cardiomyopathy show apparent massive global enlargement of the heart. Although the possibility of a pericardial effusion should be considered, in this case no effusion was seen.

Suggested Reading
Elliot LP. Chest film in myocardial ischemia resulting in left ventricular failure. In: Taveras JM, Ferrucci JT, eds. *Radiology: diagnosis-imaging-intervention.* Philadelphia: JB Lippincott, 1996;76:1–4.

Pericardial Effusion

KEY FACTS

- Pericarditis typically leads to pericardial effusions. Causes of pericarditis include neoplasia, infections (e.g., tuberculosis or viruses), rheumatic fever, radiation, and collagen vascular disease, after surgery, myocardial infarction, or in response to certain medications.

- Pericardial effusion can accompany congestive left-side heart failure, renal failure, or other systemic conditions.

- When the effusion is large, the frontal radiograph usually shows an enlarged cardiac silhouette with a "water bottle" appearance. A rapid enlargement of the silhouette should raise suspicion of a pericardial effusion.

- Occasionally seen on the lateral radiograph is displacement of the epicardial from mediastinal fat stripe by more than 2 mm. This sign, however, is present in fewer than 15% of patients with pericardial effusion.

- Echocardiography, computed tomography (CT), and magnetic resonance imaging (MRI) scanning best show pericardial effusions. Echocardiography has the advantage of portability.

- Some tissue characterization is possible with CT or MRI scanning (e.g., hemorrhagic and nonhemorrhagic effusions can be distinguished).

- Cardiac tamponade can occur when the effusion, under tension, obstructs inflow of blood to the heart. This is usually diagnosed clinically, and by echocardiography.

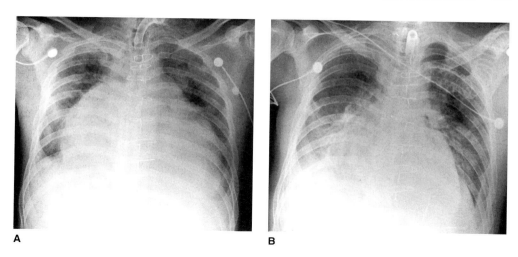

A   **B**

F I G U R E   1 9 - 2   (**A**) Anteroposterior chest radiograph of a 28-year-old-man who suffered a gunshot wound to the chest several months prior, shows a large water bottle shaped heart, which is consistent with a large pericardial effusion, related to postpericardiotomy syndrome. (**B**) Subsequent pigtail catheter drainage shows a decrease in the heart size.

Suggested Reading

Tehranzadeh J, Kelley MJ. Differential density sign of pericardial effusion. *Radiology* 1979; 133:23.

Left Ventricular Aneurysm

KEY FACTS

- Ventricular aneurysm is a sequela of a transmural myocardial infarction.
- True aneurysms contain all myocardial layers and have a wide mouth.
- False aneurysms are contained only by pericardium and are at risk for rupture.
- On chest radiographs, an abnormally convex contour is usually evident, occurring most often at the cardiac apex. The heart is usually enlarged.
- Linear calcification along the border of the left side of the heart is very suggestive of left ventricular aneurysm.
- Cross-sectional imaging can show a clot within the aneurysm.

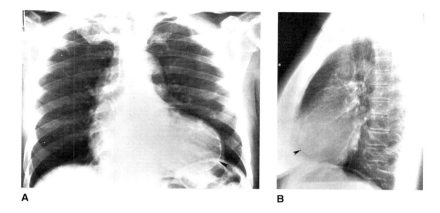

FIGURE 19-3 Frontal **(A)** and lateral **(B)** chest radiographs show a bulging left ventricular contour caused by a left ventricular aneurysm. This curvilinear calcification marginates the aneurysm (*arrowheads*), which is consistent with prior myocardial infarction.

Suggested Reading

Vlodaver Z, Coe JI, Edwards JE. True and false left ventricular aneurysms: propensity for the latter to rupture. Circulation 1975;51:567.

Calcified Pericardium from Tuberculous Pericarditis

KEY FACTS

- Calcified pericardium is a sequela of tuberculous pericarditis. More recently, viral pericarditis has become the most common cause of calcified pericardium.
- Pericardial calcification is a marker for constrictive pericarditis.
- Constrictive pericarditis causes poor ventricular diastolic filling. Patients often present with shortness of breath.
- On chest radiographs, the border of the right side of the heart may be less convex than normal.
- Computed tomography demonstrates pericardial calcification more clearly than do chest radiographs.

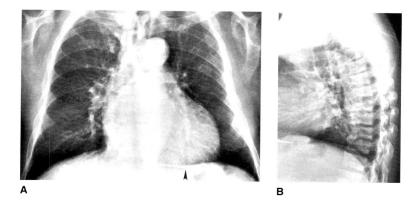

FIGURE 19-4　Posteroanterior **(A)** and lateral **(B)** chest radiographs of a patient with long-standing renal failure and uremia. PA radiograph shows thick pericardial calcification along the inferior margin of the heart (*arrowhead*). Lateral radiograph shows dense spine caused by renal osteodystrophy.

Suggested Reading

Cornell SH, Rossi NP. Radiographic findings in constrictive pericarditis. *Am J Radiol* 1968; 102:301.

Absent Left Pericardium

KEY FACTS

- Absence of the pericardium can be partial or complete, and it is nearly always found on the left.
- The partial form is occasionally associated with cardiac torsion and life-threatening symptoms such as syncope.
- The complete form is usually asymptomatic.
- On chest radiographs, the partial form shows a focal convexity in the region of the left atrial appendage. The complete form shows a shift of the heart toward the left side of the chest. Aerated lung may invaginate between the bottom of the heart and the diaphragm.
- Absence of the pericardium is well shown on coronal MRIs.

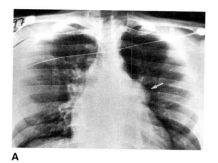
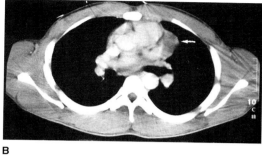

A   **B**

FIGURE 19-5   Posteroanterior chest **(A)** radiograph and CT scan **(B)** of a trauma patient show leftward bulging of the mediastinum in the region of the left atrial appendage (*arrows*), which corresponds to a partial defect in the left hemopericardium.

Suggested Reading

Nosser WK, Helmer C, Tavel ME, et al. Congenital absence of the left pericardium. *Circulation* 1970;41:469.

Cardiac Myxoma

KEY FACTS

- Myxoma is the most common primary cardiac tumor and it accounts for up to 50% of primary lesions.

- Of myxomas, 75% occur in the left atrium, 20% in the right atrium, and the remainder in the ventricles.

- In the atrium, the lesion is usually pedunculated and attached to the septum in the region of the fossa ovalis.

- During ventricular diastole, left atrial tumor may prolapse into the left ventricle.

- Patients present with valvular obstruction, embolic phenomena, and constitutional symptoms.

- The chest radiograph is usually normal. Calcified myxomas are visualized only rarely. Most project over the left atrium.

- Diagnosis is established by echocardiography, CT scan, or MRI, all of which show the mass in a cardiac chamber.

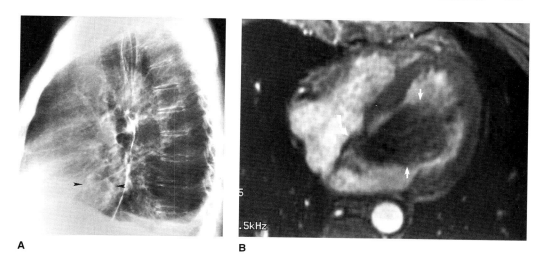

A **B**

FIGURE 19-6 (**A**) Lateral chest radiograph shows a calcified mass (*arrowheads*) projecting over the posterior heart representing a left atrial myxoma. (**B**) Axial gradient-echo MRI shows a low signal intensity mass (*arrows*). The left atrial mass is attached to the atrial septum (*curved arrow*) and has prolapsed through the mitral valve into the left ventricle.

Suggested Reading

St. John Sutton MG, Mercier LA, Guiliani ER, et al. Atrial myxomas: a review of clinical experience in 40 patients. *Mayo Clin Proc* 1980;55:371–376.

Cardiomyopathy

KEY FACTS

- Cardiomyopathies are classified as dilated, hypertrophic, or restrictive. Dilated (congestive) cardiomyopathy is the most common type.

- Dilated cardiomyopathy is often cryptogenic. Identified causes include viral infections, ischemia, metabolic diseases, collagen vascular disease, and toxins (particularly alcohol and adriamycin), and nutritional disease (beriberi).

- On chest radiography, the cardiac silhouette is enlarged and evidence may be seen of pulmonary venous hypertension caused by systolic and diastolic dysfunction. The appearance can mimic that of a pericardial effusion.

- On cross-sectional studies, the heart is markedly enlarged because of chamber dilation, not wall hypertrophy. The ventricles are of normal thickness. The ejection fraction is diminished.

- Hypertrophic cardiomyopathy is classified as obstructive or nonobstructive; the former is most important. Idiopathic hypertrophic subaortic stenosis (IHSS) is the most important entity; it leads to subaortic outflow obstruction and sudden death from associated arrhythmias.

- The chest radiograph is nonspecific in appearance; hypertrophy occurs at the expense of chamber volume. Cross-sectional techniques show marked left ventricular thickening, particularly involving the septum with nearly complete obliteration of the left ventricular cavity and outflow obstruction by the anterior leaflet of the mitral valve during systole.

- Restrictive cardiomyopathy is caused by infiltration of the heart (e.g., by amyloid, iron, or sarcoidosis), causing impairment of diastolic filling. The chest radiograph is often normal but may show evidence of pulmonary venous congestion. Cross-sectional techniques show evidence of elevated right-side heart pressure.

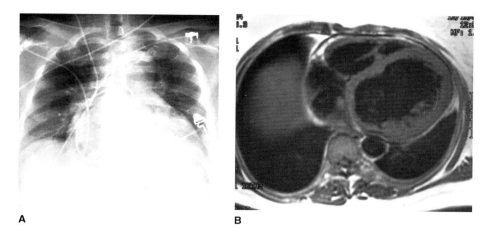

A   **B**

F I G U R E   1 9 - 7   (**A**) Posteroanterior chest radiograph shows an enlarged heart. A pulmonary arterial catheter is present. (**B**) Axial T1-weighted spin-echo MRI shows marked dilation of the left ventricle.

Suggested Reading

Goodwin JF. The frontiers of cardiomyopathy. *Br Heart J* 1982;48:1–18.

Aortic Valve Stenosis

KEY FACTS

- Aortic valve stenosis can be categorized into three groups: congenital, degenerative, and rheumatic.

  Congenital aortic stenosis usually manifests in infancy or childhood because of narrowing of a unicuspid or bicuspid aortic valve.

  Degenerative aortic stenosis can affect a bicuspid or tricuspid valve. Presentation with a bicuspid valve is usually in the fourth through sixth decades, whereas patients with degenerative involvement of a tricuspid valve present in the seventh decade or later.

  Rheumatic (see Mitral Valve Stenosis)

- Aortic stenosis causes a pressure load on the left ventricle. On chest radiography, the heart is normal in size unless left-side heart failure or associated aortic regurgitation is present. In uncomplicated cases, the pulmonary vasculature is normal.

- Calcification of the aortic valve is a suggestive finding but it is seen only in a few patients with severe aortic stenosis. A bicuspid valve is sometimes recognized by the "Mexican hat" appearance of the valve calcification.

- Another less specific finding is aorta dilation restricted to the ascending thoracic aorta, which is caused by the turbulent jet that emanates from the stenotic valve. In patients with aortic regurgitation, the ascending *and* descending aorta are enlarged.

- If congestive heart failure supervenes, the left ventricle enlarges and pulmonary venous hypertension is evident.

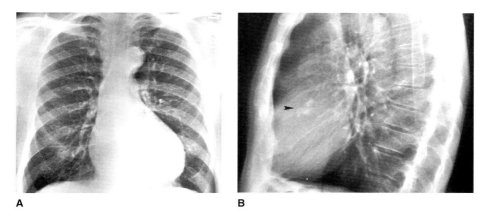

A   **B**

FIGURE 19-8   Posteroanterior (**A**) and lateral (**B**) chest radiographs of a patient with a systolic murmur. PA radiograph shows enlargement of ascending aorta and rounding of the left ventricular contour. Lateral radiograph shows calcification of the aortic valve (*arrowhead*).

Suggested Reading

Elliot LP. Chest film in aortic valve stenosis. In: Taveras JM, Ferrucci JT, eds. *Radiology: diagnosis, imaging, intervention.* Philadelphia: Lippincott–Raven Publishers, 1996.

Mitral Valve Stenosis

KEY FACTS

- Mitral valve stenosis is nearly always caused by rheumatic heart disease. Two thirds of patients are female. Symptoms may not appear for 15 to 20 years after the insult.

- Associated mitral regurgitation may be present.

- The radiographic findings of mitral valve stenosis are characteristic, and they include evidence of left atrial enlargement, manifested by a double-density along the border of the right side of the heart, uplifting of the left main bronchus, and straightening or convexity of left atrial appendage. On the lateral radiograph, posterior bulging of the left atrial contour is evident. A markedly dilated left atrium can rarely obstruct the left lower lobe bronchus and cause atelectasis. Occasionally mitral valve calcification is evident. It is important to distinguish between mitral annular calcification, which is C or J shaped, from valve calcification. Annular calcification is usually not associated with mitral stenosis.

- If the left ventricle is enlarged, substantial mitral regurgitation should be suspected.

- Invariably, evidence is seen of pulmonary venous hypertension that can include cephalization and interstitial or air–space pulmonary edema.

- Long-standing mitral stenosis leads to pulmonary arterial hypertension, manifested radiographically as enlarged central pulmonary arteries. Ultimately, high pulmonary pressures lead to right ventricle hypertrophy, tricuspid regurgitation, right-side heart dilation, and right-sided heart failure.

- A rare late complication of mitral valve stenosis is pulmonary ossification, which is caused by leeching of hemosiderin products into the interstitium (hemosiderosis) with mineral deposition and ossification. The radiographic appearance can be similar to that of multiple calcifying lung granulomas.

- Atrial fibrillation with pulmonary or systemic embolization is an associated feature.

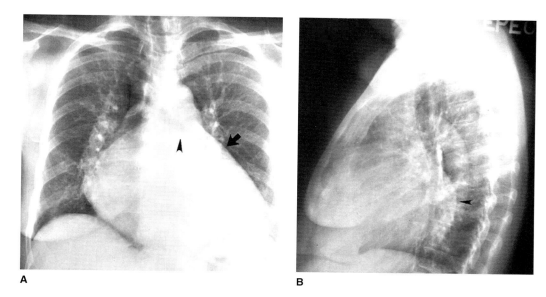

A   B

F I G U R E   1 9 - 9   Posteroanterior (PA) and lateral chest radiographs of a patient with a diastolic murmur. (**A**) PA radiograph shows enlargement of the heart and convexity of the left atrial appendage (*arrow*). The left main bronchus is uplifted (*arrowhead*). (**B**) Lateral radiograph shows cardiac enlargement with posterior convexity of the left atrium (*arrowhead*).

Suggested Reading

Chen JTT, Bahar VS, Morris JJ, et al. Correlation of roentgen findings with hemodynamic data in pure mitral stenosis. *AJR* 1968;102:280.

Atrial Septal Defect

KEY FACTS

- The most common congenital heart defect manifesting in adults is an atrial septal defect (ASD). It comprises two third of congenital heart disease treated surgically in adults. Other congenital heart lesions that occasionally manifest in adulthood include ventricular septal defect, pulmonic stenosis, and patent ductus arteriosis.

- Atrial septal defect is classified into four types: (a) ostium secundum, (b) ostium primum (associated with Down's syndrome), (c) sinus-venous (associated with partial anomalous pulmonary venous return, and (d) posteroinferior (associated with absence of the coronary sinus).

- The major hemodynamic effect of an ASD is a left-to-right shunt.

- The chest radiograph in patients with a small ASD is normal. An ASD with greater than 2:1 shunt fraction is typically pulmonary overcirculation characterized by enlarged pulmonary arteries extending more distally into the lung than normal.

- Cardiomegaly is often present. No features distinguish ASD from other left-to-right shunts in adults.

- Patients with an ASD have an increased prevalence of mitral valve prolapse, which can lead to mitral regurgitation and enlargement of the left side of the heart.

- Eventually, patients with ASD can develop Eisenmengers physiology (shunt reversal), which can sometimes be recognized on chest radiograph by enlargement of the central pulmonary arteries with more distal tapering.

- Diagnosis of the precise type of ASD requires echocardiography, angiography, or MRI.

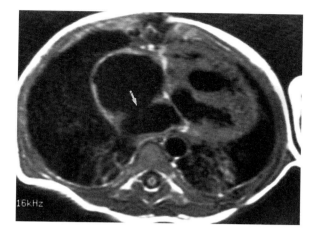

FIGURE 19-10

Axial T1-weighted spin echo MRI of a girl with pulmonary atresia shows communication between the right and left atrium (*arrow*) representing an atrial septal defect.

Suggested Reading

Green CE, Gottdiener JS, Goldstein HA. Atrial septal defect. *Semin Roentgenol* 1985;20: 214–225.

Ventricular Septal Defect

KEY FACTS

- Ventricular septal defect (VSD) is the second most common congenital heart lesion (after ASD) that occurs in adults.
- Ventricular septal defect can be classified as inlet (atrioventricular canal), muscular, perimembranous, and outlet. The perimembranous type is most common.
- The hemodynamic effect of an isolated VSD is a left-to-right shunt. Shunt extent is determined by the size of the defect and the pulmonary vascular resistance.
- The VSD found in adults is often small (Maladie de Roger).
- Many isolated VSD lesions, particularly muscular and perimembranous VSD, close spontaneously.
- Patients with VSD often develop substantial chronic elevations of pulmonary vascular resistance, manifested as pulmonary artery hypertension. The elevated pressure leads to a reversal of the left-to-right shunt (Eisenmengers physiology). At presentation, many adults have Eisenmengers physiology.
- In patients with a substantial left-to-right shunt (> 2:1), the chest radiograph shows an overcirculation pattern and left-side heart enlargement. In patients with Eisenmengers physiology, enlarged central pulmonary arteries are present with pruning of more distal arteries.
- Definitive diagnosis requires echocardiography, angiography, or MRI.

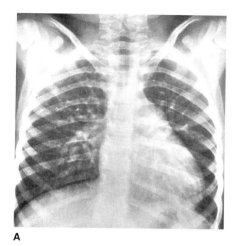

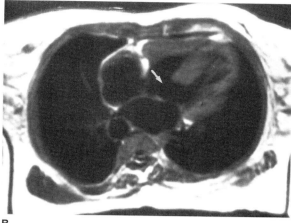

A   **B**

FIGURE 19-11   (**A**) Posteroanterior chest radiograph shows enlarged nontapering pulmonary vessels consistent with overcirculation caused by a ventricular septal defect. (**B**) Axial T1-weighted spin-echo MRI in a different patient shows a defect in the membranous portion (*arrow*) of the ventricular septum. This patient had tetralogy of Fallot.

Suggested Reading
Didier D, Higgins CB. Identification and localization of ventricular septal defect by gated magnetic resonance imaging. *Am J Cardiol* 1986;57:1363–1368.

20   The Hila

Bilateral Hilar Enlargement

KEY FACTS

- Common causes of bilateral hilar enlargement include metastatic disease such as small-cell carcinoma, lymphoma (see Chap. 14), infectious granulomatous disease including tuberculosis and fungi, and sarcoidosis. Vascular causes are also common, including primary and secondary pulmonary artery hypertension from a variety of underlying diseases (see Chap. 18).

- Rarer causes of hilar enlargement include Castleman's disease, angioimmunoblastic lymphadenopathy, silicosis, berylliosis, and phenytoin therapy.

- Hilar enlargement is often asymmetric, particularly in cases of metastatic disease, lymphomas, or infectious granulomatous disease.

- Symmetric hilar adenopathy is common in sarcoidosis.

- Calcified hilar lymphadenopathy is common in patients with previous granulomatous infection, silicosis, and sarcoidosis. An eggshell pattern of calcification can occur in silicosis, sarcoidosis, and treated lymphoma.

- Dense contrast enhancement in lymph nodes may occur in the hyaline-vascular type of Castleman's disease.

- Tuberculous mediastinitis can show a low density central region after contrast-enhanced CT scan. Low density lymph nodes can also occur in lymphoma and metastatic lymphadenopathy.

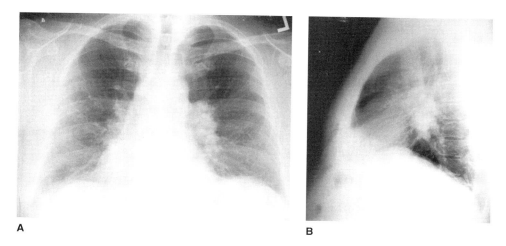

FIGURE 20-1 Posteroanterior **(A)** and lateral **(B)** chest radiographs of a 46-year-old man, who has worked for many years in the nuclear power industry, show bilateral hilar masses strongly suggestive of adenopathy. Although this appearance is typical of sarcoidosis, this patient had occupational beryllium exposure and proven berylliosis, which is radiographically indistinguishable from sarcoidosis.

Suggested Reading

Mediastinal and hilar disorders. In: Armstrong P, Wilson AG, Dee P, et al., eds. *Imaging of diseases of the chest*, 2nd ed. St. Louis: Mosby, 1995;16:713–816.

Sarcoidosis

KEY FACTS

- Saroidosis is a multisystem disorder characterized by the presence of noncaseating granulomas. Although sarcoidosis can involve virtually any organ, intrathoracic involvement is seen in up to 90% of the cases.

- A radiographic classification can be used to help prognosticate the chances of spontaneous remission.

  Stage 0 = Normal chest radiograph

  Stage 1 = Mediastinal and hilar lymphadenopathy

  Stage 2 = Mediastinal and hilar lymphadenopathy with lung parenchymal infiltrates

  Stage 3 = Parenchymal infiltrates only

  Stage 4 = Lung fibrosis

- Radiographically, symmetric bilateral hilar lymphadenopathy accompanied by right paratracheal adenopathy is typical of sarcoidosis, and this is termed "Garland's triad." Up to 10% of patients have asymmetric hilar lymphadenopathy. Pulmonary parenchymal findings include reticulonodular or miliary shadowing and alveolar opacities that may be nondescript or may form ill-defined nodules.

- Enlargement of mediastinal and hilar lymph nodes is usually diffuse, discrete, and symmetric. Lymph nodes can calcify.

- Approximately 25% of patients develop pulmonary fibrosis. The typical radiograph appearance is course linear opacities extending from the hila into the middle and upper lung zones. In end-stage sarcoidosis, traction bronchiectasis can be seen adjacent to peribronchial fibrosis. This can show cystic changes on the chest radiograph. Similar findings can sometimes result from emphysematous bullae that arise from adjacent areas of fibrosis. Both bronchiectasis and bullae can become colonized by fungi, forming a mycetoma (see Chap. 12).

- So-called "alveolar sarcoidosis" represents extension of granlomatous infiltration from the interstitium to the alveolar space. Alveolar sarcoid can present radiographically as fluffy infiltrates with air bronchograms that can simulate pneumonia, pulmonary masses, or metastasis.

- High resolution CT scan findings of sarcoidosis within the lung parenchyma include small nodules, interlobular septal thickening, and, ultimately, traction bronchiectasis. The changes tend to be distributed along bronchovascular bundles and in a subpleural location.

- Unusual thoracic manifestations of sarcoidosis include airways disease, pleural disease, and cavitary lung masses. True cavitation in sarcoid is rare and is thought to occur when ischemic necrosis from granulomatous vasculitis of the pulmonary arteries leads to necrosis and liquefaction of confluent sarcoid granulomas.

- Atypical nodal locations may be evident on CT including the anterior mediastinum, axilla, internal mammary chains, and retrocrural regions. Nodal calcification ultimately occurs in as many as 20% of patients.

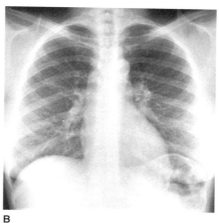

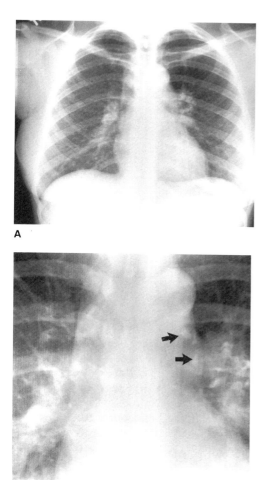

FIGURE 20-2

(A) Posteroanterior chest radiograph of a 31-year-old-woman shows mild bilateral hilar enlargement. **(B)** Twelve years later, bilateral hilar enlargement remains. Note there are now calcified lymph nodes best seen in the aorticopulmonary window, and also seen better in the close-up **(C)** (*arrows*).

(continued)

Sarcoidosis (Continued)

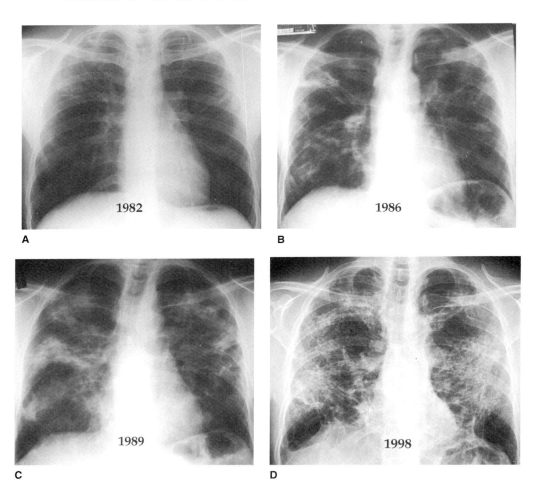

FIGURE 20-3 (**A**) Posteroanterior chest radiograph of a 29-year-old-man with sarcoidosis shows very mild patchy areas of lung fibrosis and no adenopathy (1982). (**B**) From 1986, patchy lung fibrosis has progressed with a somewhat nodular appearance. (**C**) In 1989 the nodular fibrotic masses have progressed further. (**D**) Finally in 1998, an appearance of end-stage lung fibrosis exists, with traction bronchiectasis seen as cystic changes on the chest radiograph.

Suggested Reading

Kuhlman JE, Fishman EK, Hamper UM, et al. The computed tomographic spectrum of thoracic sarcoidosis. *Radiographics* 1989;9:449–466.

Section 4

THE CHEST WALL, PLEURA, AND DIAPHRAGM

21 Chest Wall Abnormalities

Pectus Deformity

KEY FACTS

- Two types of pectus deformity are seen: pectus carinatum and pectus excavatum.

- Pectus excavatum, also called a "funnel chest deformity," is a depression of the sternum that displaces the heart backward and to the left. It can have physiologic significance by impairing peak physical performance; it is often corrected surgically.

- The chest radiograph shows the heart shifted to the left. The border of the right side of the heart can be obscured by the thoracic spine. The reoriented right chest wall and compressed lung tissue can simulate a right middle lobe pneumonia. The sternal depression is easily seen on the lateral view.

- Pectus carinatum, also called a "pigeon breast deformity," is a cosmetic (and potentially psychologic) problem only.

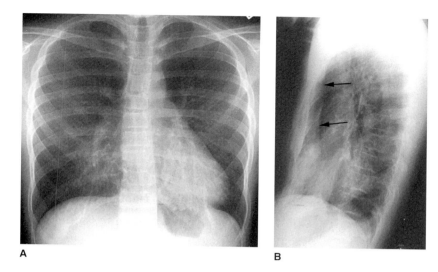

A   B

FIGURE 21-1   Posteroanterior **(A)** and lateral **(B)** chest radiographs of a 20-year-old man show a posterior depression of the sternum that displaces the heart backward and to the left (*arrows*). The border of the right side of the heart is obscured by the thoracic spine. Note the opacity along the border of the right side of the heart that simulates right middle lobe pneumonia. No corresponding opacity is seen on the lateral view.

Suggested Reading

Kuhlman JE, Bouchardy L, Fishman EK, et al. CT and MR imaging evaluation of chest wall disorders. *Radiographics* 1994;14:571–595.

Actinomycosis

K E Y   F A C T S

- Actinomycosis is caused by a gram-positive anaerobic bacteria. *A. israelii* is the most common causative organism.
- Sulfur granules, so named because of their yellow color, form within tissues.
- The organism is a normal colonizer of the oral flora.
- The lungs are involved in 10% of actinomycosis cases. Other sites of involvement include the uterus, often related to intrauterine devices, and the gastrointestinal tract.
- Aspiration of oral contents permits entry of the organism into the lungs.
- On chest radiographs, actinomycosis appears as a nonspecific, nonsegmental area of consolidation which may be masslike.
- Complications of pulmonary actinomycosis include empyema and chest wall invasion, with sinus track formation.
- In cases with chest wall invasion, the ribs often show periostitis rather than frank destruction.

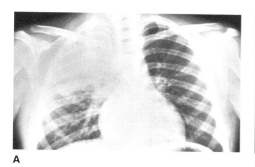
A

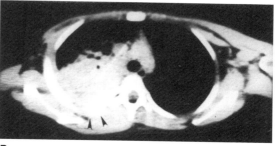
B

FIGURE 21-2   (**A**) Posteroanterior chest radiograph of a teenage boy shows dense consolidation in the right upper lung. (**B**) On CT scan, invasion of the posterior chest wall (*arrowheads*) is seen.

Suggested Reading

Flynn MW, Felson B. The roentgen manifestations of thoracic actinomycosis. *AJR* 1970;110: 707–716.

Dermatomyositis

KEY FACTS

- Dermatomyositis is characterized by proximal muscle weakness and a violaceous skin rash. Polymyositis is similar but it spares the skin.
- Diagnosis is based on elevation of serum muscle enzymes and muscle biopsy.
- Coexistent malignant disease occurs in approximately 15% of patients. Tumors of the lung, ovary, breast, and gastrointestinal track predominate.
- Most patients have normal chest radiographs. Interstitial lung fibrosis occurs in about 5% of patients and as with other interstitial fibroses most often involves the lung bases.
- Subcutaneous calcification, which can be quite striking, can affect the extremities, abdominal wall, pelvis, or chest wall.
- These calcifications are often fine, reticular, or streaky early in the disease and become coarser as the disease progresses.

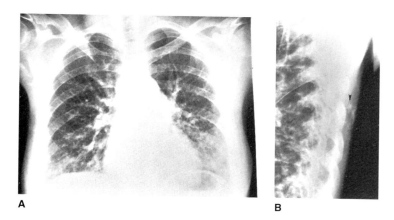

A   B

FIGURE 21-3   (**A**) Posteroanterior chest radiograph shows coarsening of the interstitial markings at the lung bases. (**B**) Coned-down lateral radiograph of the posterior chest shows calcifications in the chest wall (*arrowhead*).

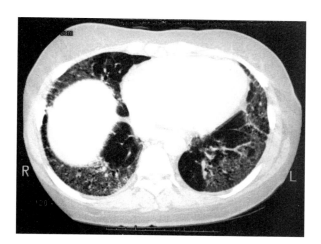

FIGURE 21-4

High resolution CT scan of a patient with dermatomyositis shows the typical changes of basilar interstitial pulmonary fibrosis including thickened septal lines, parenchymal bands, distortion of lung architecture, and subpleural honeycombing.

Suggested Reading

Ozonoff MB, Flynn FJ. Roentgenologic features of dermatomyositis of childhood. *AJR* 1973; 118:206–212.

Osteochondroma

KEY FACTS

- Osteochondroma is a histologically benign exostosis of bone that contains a cartilage cap.
- The most common location of the lesion is the metaphysis of a long bone, especially around the knee.
- Osteochondroma is the most common cartilaginous or osteogenic neoplasm of the chest wall.
- In the chest, the ribs and scapula are most often affected, although other bones can be involved.
- Less than 1% of cases undergo malignant degeneration to chondrosarcoma.
- Interval growth of a previously stable lesion or a lesion with a large soft-tissue component are features that suggest malignant degeneration.

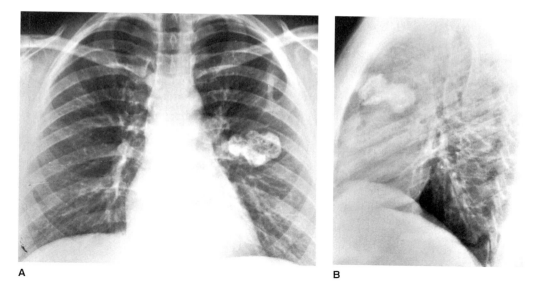

FIGURE 21-5 Posteroanterior (**A**) and lateral (**B**) chest radiographs show a densely calcified lesion that originates from the left anterior third rib. (Courtesy of Robert Pugatch, M.D., Baltimore, MD.)

Suggested Reading
Marcove RC, Huvos AG. Cartilaginous tumors of the ribs. *Cancer* 1971;27:794.

Neurofibromatosis

KEY FACTS

- Neurofibromatosis type 1 (von Recklinghausen's disease) is transmitted as an autosomal dominant trait and has multiple thoracic manifestations.

- Intrathoracic lesions include mediastinal and paraspinal neurogenic tumors, pheochromocytomas, and interstitial lung fibrosis, which consist of both basilar reticular and apical bullous changes.

- Changes of the thoracic cage include kyphoscoliosis, often with sharp angulation, and rib dysplasias, which may cause "ribbon" ribs due to a modeling deformity.

- Dural ectasia is another manifestation of neurofibromatosis, which may be caused by neurogenic tumors with both intra and extracanalicular components (dumbbell tumors) and lateral meningoceles.

- Cutaneous findings are frequent, consisting of a variety of mesenchymal tumors, particularly neurofibromas and schwannomas (fibroma molluscum).

- On chest radiography, the skin lesions project over the lungs and can be misdiagnosed as parenchymal nodules. Error can be avoided by looking for nodules projecting over soft tissues. The lateral chest radiograph often allows localization of the nodules to the anterior or posterior chest wall.

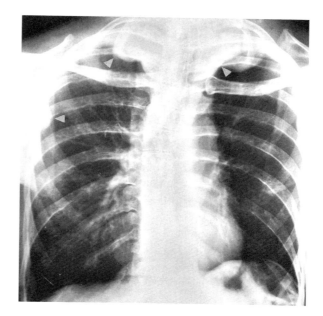

FIGURE 21-6
Posteroanterior chest radiograph shows extrapleural biapical and bilateral chest wall soft-tissue masses (*arrowheads*) corresponding to multiple neurofibromas.

Suggested Reading

Klatte EC, Franken EA, Smith JA. The radiographic spectrum in neurofibromatosis. *Semin Roentgenol* 1976;11:17–33.

Skeletal Metastases

KEY FACTS

- Metastases affect the axial skeleton, which includes the ribs and thoracic spine, in up to 60% of cases.
- Most metastatic disease spreads hematogenously. Metastases can bypass the lungs and directly reach the spine by way of Batson's plexus of veins.
- Common sites of origin of osteolytic metastases to the skeleton include the lung, breast, kidney, and thyroid. Breast cancer has the highest frequency of metastasis to bone.
- Prostate carcinoma is the most common source of osteoblastic metastases. Other primary tumors that cause osteoblastic metastases include mucinous carcinomas and hematologic malignancy.
- Radiographically, osteolytic bone metastases are visualized as focal areas of lucency, and they are often expansile. Renal and thyroid bone metastases have the greatest tendency to cause expansile lesions. Osteoblastic bone metastases are seen as areas of increased bone density. The lesions, which can affect the ribs, spine, or shoulder girdle, are often multiple.
- Radionuclide bone scanning is useful to show multiplicity of lesions, including lesions that may not be evident on a skeletal survey.
- Computed tomography or MRI also can be useful to show metastatic disease, particularly if it involves the spine.
- The main differential diagnosis for osteolytic metastases is multiple myeloma. For osteoblastic metastases, a wide variety of conditions can appear similar, including renal osteodystrophy, Paget's disease, myelofibrosis, and osteopetrosis.

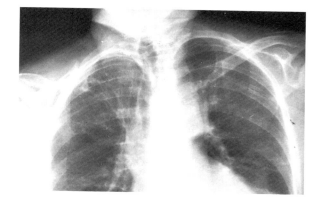

F I G U R E   2 1 - 7
Posteroanterior chest radiograph of a woman with metastatic breast cancer shows destruction of the right clavicle.

Suggested Reading

Krishnamurthy GT, Tubis M, Hiss J, Blahd WH. Distribution pattern of metastatic bone disease. *JAMA* 1977;237:2504–2506.

Congenital Rib Anomalies

KEY FACTS

- Congenital anomalies of the ribs are quite common, and most are asymptomatic.
- Bifid or fused ribs are readily recognized on chest radiography by their characteristic appearance.
- Cervical ribs occur in 0.5% of patients, and they are more common in women. In a small proportion of patients, the supernumerary ribs compress the brachial plexus or subclavian vessels, causing symptoms of thoracic outlet syndrome.
- On chest radiography, the C-7 vertebral body bears the extra rib or ribs.
- When thoracic outlet syndrome is present and the radiograph shows a cervical rib or ribs, angiography or MRI is often confirmatory.
- A rare congenital anomaly of the ribs is an intrathoracic rib. This supernumerary rib arises in the thorax, more often on the right. It can originate from the vertebral body or another rib. The intrathoracic rib usually has a more caudal course than normal. An intrathoracic rib is typically asymptomatic.

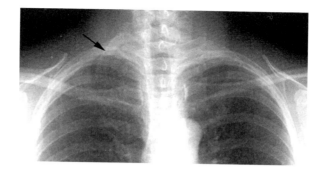

FIGURE 21-8

Frontal view of the upper chest shows a unilateral, right-sided cervical rib (*arrow*).

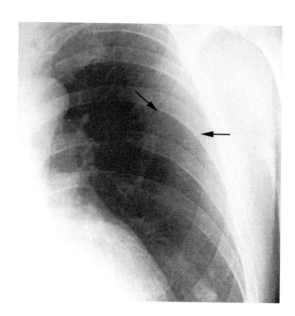

FIGURE 21-9

Frontal view of the left chest shows a bifid left anterior rib (*arrows*). This is an asymptomatic normal variant.

Suggested Reading

Fisher MS. Eve's rib. *Radiology* 1981;140:841.

Lung Hernia

KEY FACTS

- Lung hernia is a protrusion of the lung with visceral and parietal pleura through a defect in the thoracic cage.
- Lung hernias are classified by location and cause. They occur at the lung apices, diaphragm, or chest wall, and are either congenital or acquired secondary to trauma, chest wall neoplasms, or infection.
- Spontaneous lung hernias have also been reported in weight lifters, wind instrument musicians, and patients with chronic cough.
- Most cases are traumatic in origin and involve the thoracic wall.
- Most apical lung hernias occur in children and they are congenital.
- Lung hernias can be missed unless the x-ray beam is at a true tangent to the hernia. CT confirms the extent and anatomy of the injury.
- Most lung hernias are asymptomatic and can be treated with a truss. Operative repair is indicated for persistent pain, incarceration, or strangulation. Currently the chosen method of repair consists of closing the defect with a GorTex patch.

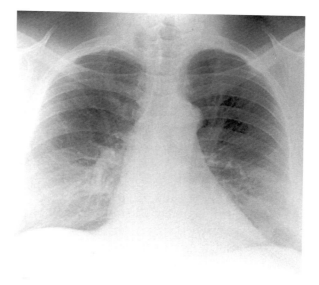

FIGURE 21-10

Posteroanterior chest radiograph of a 55-year-old man shows an incidental right apical lung hernia. Note the lucency at the right lung apex, just lateral to the tracheal air column.

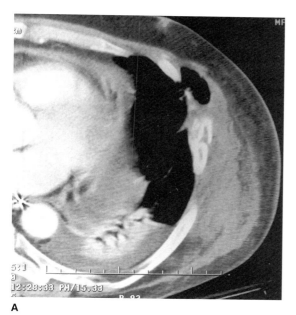

A

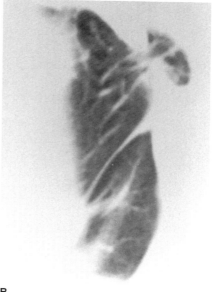

B

FIGURE 21-11   Computed tomography scan of a 71-year-old woman who suffered severe blunt trauma to her left torso with a ruptured left hemidiaphragm, multiple left rib fractures, lung contusion, and splenic laceration. A routine chest radiograph 4 days after injury showed a new lucency in the left lateral chest wall (not shown). CT scan soft-tissue window (**A**) shows an abnormal air collection extending through the chest wall. (**B**) The lung window better characterizes the normal lung tissue herniating through the post-traumatic intercostal space defect.

Suggested Reading

Bhalla M, Leitman BS, Forcade C, et al. Lung hernia: radiographic features. *AJR* 1990;154: 51–53.

Extrapleural Lipoma

KEY FACTS

- Extrapleural lipomas arise from adipose tissue in the extrapleural space or more deeply in the chest wall.
- This lesion is the most common benign tumor of the chest wall and is typically well encapsulated.
- Most lipomas are asymptomatic, but they are often bulky lesions that can protrude through the ribs and produce a palpable lesion.
- On chest radiography, lesions that are in an extrapleural location often have characteristics of a pleural lesion (i.e., they are often peripheral and one margin of the lesion is well-defined, whereas the opposite margin is indistinct).
- Small lipomas that are extracostal are usually not visible on chest radiography.
- Computed tomography scanning is diagnostic and shows a well-defined uniformly fat attenuation lesion. Occasionally, some linear strands of higher density are found. If greater quantities of soft-tissue density are admixed, a well-differentiated liposarcoma should be considered. Many small chest wall lipomas are found incidentally and are of no clinical significance.
- On MRI, lipomas characteristically show high signal intensity on T1-weighted images and somewhat lower signal intensity on T2-weighted images. Fat suppressed sequences are diagnostic.

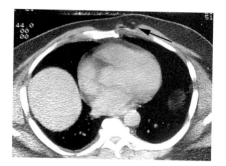

FIGURE 21-12

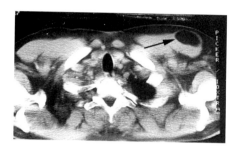

FIGURE 21-13

FIGURES 21-12, 21-13, and 21-14
Computed tomography scans of three different patients show three different incidentally found chest wall lipomas. Note that they are typically well-defined and of fat attenuation.

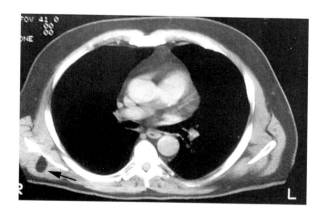

Suggested Reading

Omell GH, Anderson LS, Bramson RT. Chest wall tumors. *Radiol Clin North Am* 1973;11: 197–214.

22   **Pleural Diseases**

Pleural Effusion

KEY FACTS

- Pleural fluid normally acts as an adhesive between the parietal and visceral pleura, helping to keep the lung inflated under the force of its own elastic recoil, and also acting as a lubricant.
- Pleural fluid is continuously produced and resorbed by the parietal pleura.
- A pleural effusion is any abnormal accumulation of fluid of any kind, be it blood, transudate, chyle, and so forth, in the pleural space.
- Upright chest radiographs can reliably detect effusions of more than 100 mL. Look for blunting of the posterior costophrenic angles on the lateral chest radiograph. Supine chest radiographs may not show even large effusions.
- Lateral decubitus radiographs will quickly and easily determine if any pleural fluid is free flowing. If not free flowing, consider loculations or solid thickening. Always obtain *both* decubitus views, because one never knows which view will be most helpful.
- The size of larger pleural effusions can be *estimated* as follows. Divide the hemithorax into thirds. Those fluid collections filling a third of the hemithorax are *about* 1 L; two thirds, 2 L; "white out," about 3 L. On a lateral decubitus view, pleural effusion size can be estimated as 400 mL/cm in the midpoint of the effusion. Remember, these are "guesstimates" that help the clinician, especially when a thorocentesis is indicated.
- Transudative effusions are noninflammatory; they are caused by congestive heart failure and hypoproteinemic states such as liver cirrhosis and nephrotic syndrome.
- Exudative (parapneumonic) effusions, which are caused by pleural inflammation or impaired lymphatic drainage, are most commonly seen with malignancy and infection, although many possible diagnoses exist. Exudative effusions occur in approximately 50% of all pneumonias. Those caused by infection are often inflammatory reactions and do not necessarily contain organisms. Malignant effusions can be caused by direct pleural invasion, hematogenous spread indicating metastatic disease, or lymphatic obstruction.
- Exudative pleural effusions associated with an infection can be either uncomplicated parapneumonic effusions; complicated parapneumonic effusions, indicating a later fibropurulent stage; or frank empyemas. Rarely, loculated effusions can have more than one type.
- Other relatively common causes of pleural effusions include pancreatitis, collagen-vascular diseases, and pulmonary embolism.
- With ultrasonography, exudates are echogenic, the pleura may be thickened, and septations can be seen.
- Computed tomography (CT) scanning is much more effective in showing the size, distribution, extent, and associated findings or underlying cause, than the chest radiograph. With exudative effusions, look for pleural thickening, extrapleural fat thickening, and pleural contrast enhancement. CT scanning can show a split-pleura sign. Normally, the thin visceral and parietal pleura cannot be distinguished as two separate structures on CT

scanning. With a complicated pleural effusion or empyema, the fluid separates or "splits" the thickened and contrast-enhancing pleural layers.

- A number of different chest radiographic appearances of pleural effusions can be seen. See the accompanying figures.

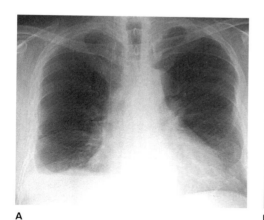

A

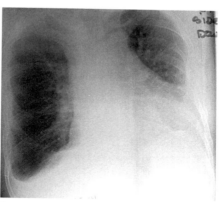

B

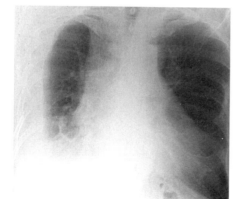

C

FIGURE 22-1

(**A**) Upright anteroposterior chest radiograph of a 37-year-old man with chronic liver disease shows blunting of the right costophrenic angle, typical of a small right pleural effusion. (**B**) Left-side down lateral decubitus chest radiograph shows no left pleural effusion, the right costophrenic angle almost completely clears, and no underlying right lung parenchymal disease is seen. (**C**) The right-side down lateral decubitus chest radiograph shows the right pleural effusion is free flowing and measures approximately 2 cm (approximately 800 mL in volume). It is also important to assess the lung parenchyma underneath the effusion; always get both decubitus views.

(continued)

Pleural Effusion (Continued)

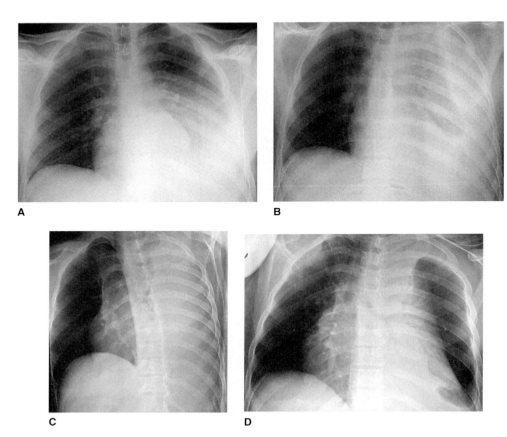

FIGURE 22-2   Semi-upright (**A**), supine (**B**), left-side down lateral decubitus (**C**), and right-side down (**D**) lateral decubitus chest radiographs of a 21-year-old man with abdominal trauma show four different appearances for this same large, mobile left pleural effusion. It is important to know the position of the patient at the time the radiograph was obtained for accurate interpretation. Also, it is very important to have consistent positioning from one examination to the next, to accurately interpret the amount of fluid within the pleural space.

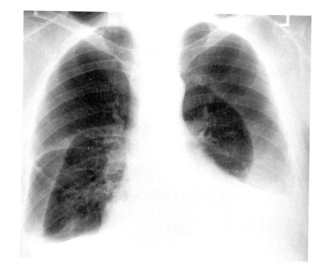

FIGURE 22-3

Semi-upright anteroposterior chest radiograph of a 60-year-old man shows
bilateral pleural effusions tracking into
both major fissures, which are likely to
be incomplete fissures. Do not confuse
the normal aerated lung, medially, for
abnormal air collections.

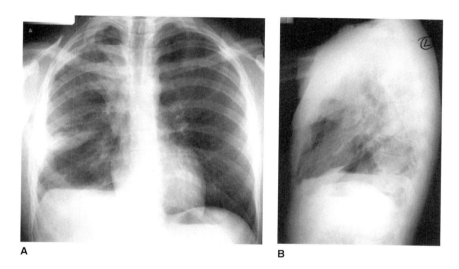

A   **B**

FIGURE 22-4   Posteroanterior **(A)** and lateral **(B)** chest radiographs of a 42-year-old man show a
subpulmonic right pleural effusion. Note the shouldering or lateral displacement of
the normal mid-diaphragmatic hump. Fluid tracking into the right minor fissure is
also seen.

(continued)

Pleural Effusion (Continued)

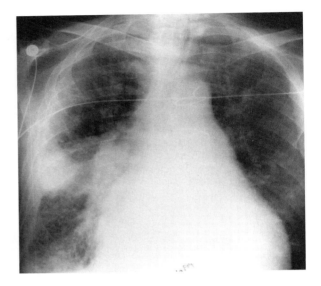

FIGURE 22-5
Anteroposterior chest radiograph of a 72-year-old man shows cardiomegaly and a right pleural effusion. Note the effusion tracks into the minor fissure, which on occasion can appear masslike, as in this case. This tumor vanished in 1 day after medical therapy for congestive heart failure.

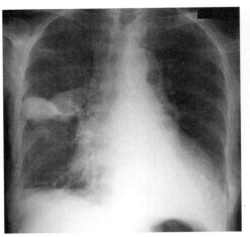

A

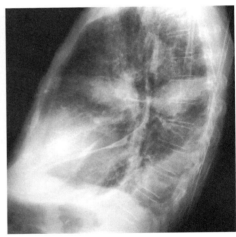

B

FIGURE 22-6   Posteroanterior (**A**) and lateral (**B**) chest radiographs of an 82-year-old man show cardiomegaly and a right pleural effusion, best seen on the lateral view. Note the effusion also tracks into both the major and minor fissures. These fluid collections can appear masslike, but they usually have a typical elliptic shape.

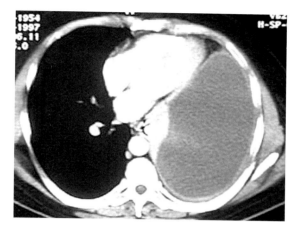

FIGURE 22-7

Computed tomography scan of a 20-year-old man with a positive purified protein derivative (PPD) and a chest radiograph showing a large left lung opacity, shows a large left pleural effusion with complete collapse of the left lung. Note some thickening and enhancement of the pleura. This was tuberculous pleurisy. The primary lung parenchymal disease is often not visible.

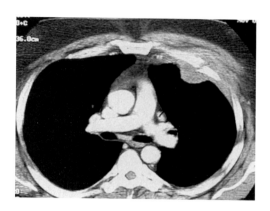

FIGURE 22-8

Computed tomography scan through the midchest shows an obvious *extra*pleural hematoma around an anterior rib fracture. A loculated pleural fluid collection is not distinguishable.

Suggested Reading

Aquino SL, Webb WR, Gushiken BJ. Pleural exudates and transudates: diagnosis with contrast-enhanced CT. *Radiology* 1994;192:803–808.

Pneumothorax

KEY FACTS

- Pneumothorax denotes the presence of air within the pleural space.
- Pneumothorax is classified as spontaneous or traumatic. Spontaneous pneumothorax can be further grouped as primary, indicating no evident inciting event, or secondary, characterized by underlying disease.
- Causes of traumatic pneumothorax are most often iatrogenic and include sequela of central line placement and mechanical ventilation. Penetrating trauma is another common cause.
- Primary spontaneous pneumothorax is most common in young men with a smoking history. A slight right-sided predilection is reported. It is usually caused by a ruptured apical bleb.
- Secondary spontaneous pneumothorax is caused by a variety of infections (e.g., pneumocystis pneumonia), neoplasms (e.g., sarcomas), interstitial lung disease, and processes characterized by airflow obstruction (e.g., asthma).
- On erect radiographs, pleural air rises to the apical and lateral parts of the hemithorax. Pneumothorax manifests as a pleural line beyond which no lung markings are present. Underlying parenchymal disease may be evident.
- In supine patients, pleural air collects anteromedially and in a subpulmonic location and may be difficult to visualize. If uncertainty exists, a lateral decubitus radiograph with the affected side superior may be valuable.
- A CT scan provides a more accurate assessment of the size of a pneumothorax and shows underlying parenchymal disease optimally; high resolution CT may define a small apical bleb as the cause of a primary spontaneous pneumothorax.
- Do not try to guess a percentage; this is notoriously inaccurate. It is best just to describe the actual, measurable pleural separation; for example, "8 mm of apical pleural separation" as seen in Fig. 22-9. This approach allows anyone to form an accurate mental picture of the size of the pneumothorax.
- We recommend *not* obtaining chest radiographs at end exhalation. Very low lung volumes can make it somewhat easier to detect a very small pneumothorax, but these views are more often misinterpreted as showing new congestive heart failure or pulmonary edema when compared with full inspiration radiographs. We feel that it is not worth the possible confusion.
- With an otherwise normal pleural space, without pleural adhesions, air collects in the most non–gravity-dependent location in the hemithorax. Obviously, this varies depending on the patient's position. In upright patients, free pleural air will collect over the lung apices, but in supine-positioned patients, free pleural air collects in the anterior, inferior pleural space, down by the hemidiaphragms. When these pneumothoraces are large, in supine-positioned patients, they are seen as the deep sulcus sign.
- The size of a pneumothorax can be vastly underestimated on supine radiographs, or even remain undetected.
- Because knowing patient inclination is so important, portable chest radiographs should always be marked as to patient position. The

technologist can mark the films by hand or use one of several types of gravity or inclination markers available in the marketplace.

- Pneumothoraces can collect in more unusual locations (e.g., medially), and they can be confused with other abnormalities such as aeroespohagus or pneumomediastinum.

- Skin folds and chest tube tracks can mimic a pneumothorax.

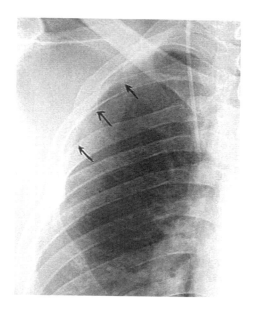

FIGURE 22-9

Upright anteroposterior chest radiograph obtained from a patient shortly after placement of a right central venous catheter shows a typical small right pneumothorax, with 8 mm of apical pleural separation (*arrows*). These small pneumothoraces can be difficult to detect, and diligence, along with proper collimation of extraneous light, is usually required to detect them.

(continued)

Pneumothorax (Continued)

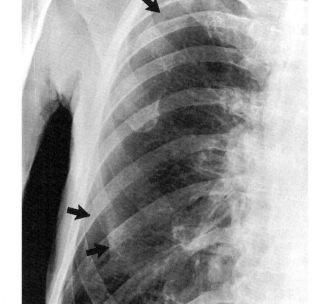

FIGURE 22-10

Upright anteroposterior chest radiograph obtained from a patient with a spontaneous pneumothorax shows a typical small right pneumothorax (*upper two arrows*) and a skin fold (*lower arrow*) as a mimic of a pneumothorax. The skin fold does not form a sharp pleural line, but, in this case, it forms a gradation of gray that fades out medially and a sharp black Mach line laterally.

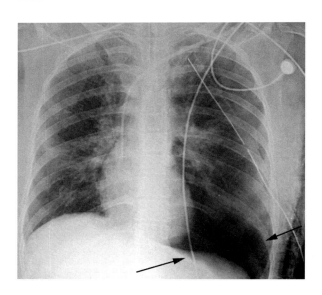

FIGURE 22-11

Anteroposterior supine chest radiograph of a patient with diffuse lung injury shows a deep sulcus sign on the left (*arrows*), despite a chest tube in place. The pneumothorax often extends off the film.

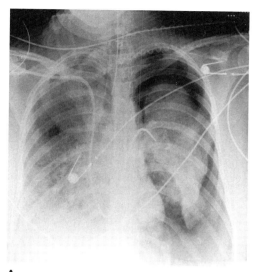
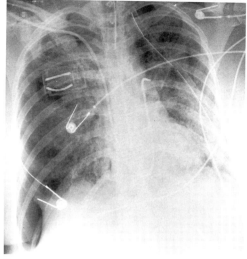

A

B

FIGURE 22-12 (A) Supine anteroposterior chest radiograph of a 34 year-old woman with acute respiratory distress syndrome (ARDS) and very high positive end-expiratory pressures, shows a large left pneumothorax. (B) Repeat examination, 2 hours later after left chest tube placement shows evacuation of the left pneumothorax, but a new, large right pneumothorax. Both views show examples of the deep sulcus sign.

(continued)

Pneumothorax (Continued)

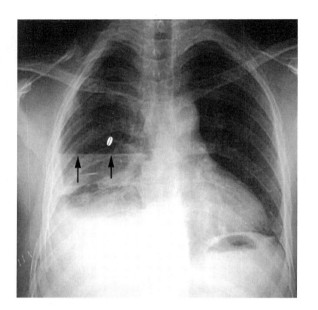

FIGURES 22-13 and 22-14

Chest radiographs from two patients with hydropneumothoraces. Sometimes the air–fluid level (*arrows* in 22-13 and *arrowheads* in 22-14A) can be easier to see than the actual pleural line (22-14**B**, *arrows*), as in these cases.

FIGURE 22-14

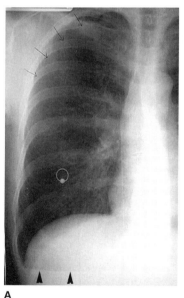

A

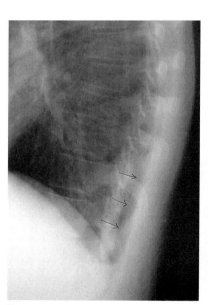

B

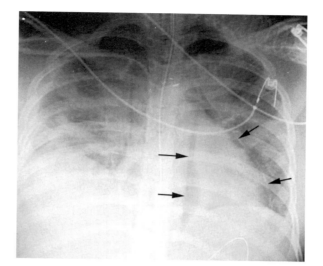

FIGURE 22-15

Supine anteroposterior chest radiograph of a patient who suffered multiple trauma shows a medial pneumothorax (*arrows*). This should not be confused with air in the esophagus or pneumomediastinum.

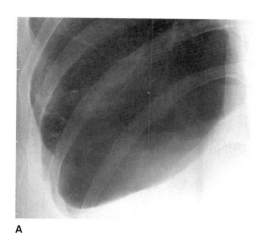

A

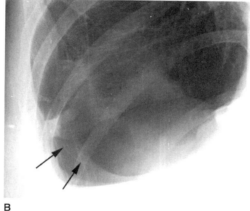

B

FIGURES 22-16A, 22-16B, and 22-17

When bullous lung disease is present, it can be very difficult to determine the presence or absence of a pneumothorax. Look for the double wall sign, with air on both sides of the wall of a bulla, evident on chest radiographs and CT scanning, as shown in these two patients (*arrows*). *Arrowheads* in Fig. 22-17 indicate paraseptal emphysema.

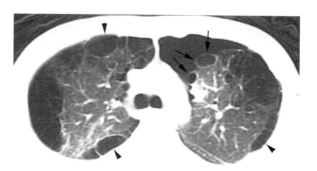

FIGURE 22-17

(continued)

Pneumothorax (Continued)

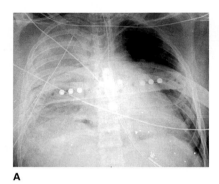

A

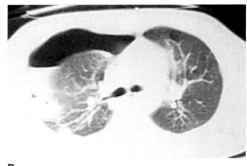

B

FIGURE 22-18   (**A**) Supine anteroposterior chest radiograph of a patient who suffered a shotgun wound shows what appears to be a large right pleural fluid collection, despite a right chest tube. The left lung appears normal. (**B**) CT scan obtained shortly after the radiograph shows a large right hydropneumothorax; the large pneumothorax was not evident on the radiograph.

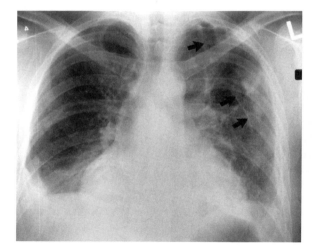

FIGURE 22-19

Posteroanterior chest radiograph of a 34-year-old man who was treated with a chest tube for a pneumothorax suffered after a motor vehicle accident shows a left chest tube track (*arrows*), evident after tube removal.

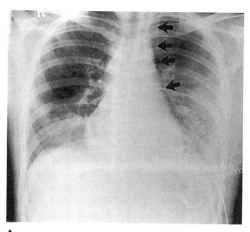
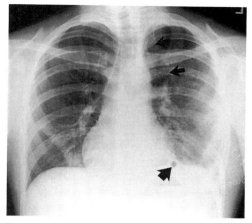

A   B

FIGURE 22-20 (**A**) Anteroposterior (AP) chest radiograph of a 27-year-old man after a left chest tube was removed shows a left chest tube track (*arrows*). Note the remaining left chest tube. (**B**) AP chest radiograph after the second chest tube was removed now shows two left chest tube tracks, the lower track is seen end-on (*arrows*). These should not be confused with pneumothoraces.

Suggested Readings

Greene R, McLoud TC, Stark P. Pneumothorax. *Semin Roentgenol* 1977;12:313–325.

Knisely BL, Kuhlman JE. Radiographic and CT imaging of complex pleural disease. *Crit Rev Diagn Imaging* 1997;38:1–58.

Extrapleural Fat

KEY FACTS

- Extrapleural fat is a benign condition in which adipose tissue may be deposited in multiple locations.
- Patients who are obese or who are receiving steroid treatments are prone to forming extrapleural fat.
- Extrapleural fat can radiographically resemble diffuse pleural thickening caused by pathologic processes such as pleural tumor or empyema.
- Radiographically, extrapleural fat is found most often between the fourth and eighth rib and extends laterally from the anterior axillary line to the angles of the ribs.
- Computed tomography scan best shows the fatty nature of the extrapleural collection.
- In addition to pathologic causes, the differential diagnosis of apparent radiographic extrapleural fat includes rib companion shadows and silhouetting by the serratus anterior muscle.

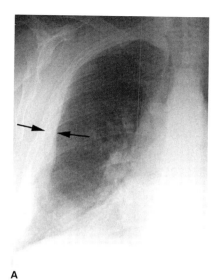

A

FIGURE 22-21

(A) Frontal chest radiograph of a 58-year-old man shows about 1 cm of "pleural thickening" (*arrows*) that is nonspecific, but could represent pleural fibrosis, loculated fluid, extrapleural fat, tumor, or hematoma. (B, C) CT scans obtained through the area in question shows the pleural opacity (*arrows*) is a focal deposition of extrapleural fat.

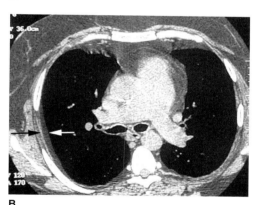

B

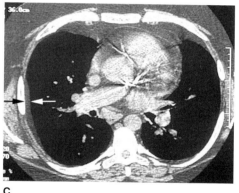

C

Suggested Reading

Sargent EN, Boswell WD, Ralls PW, et al. Subpleural fat pads in patients exposed to asbestos: distinction from non-calcified pleural plaques. *Radiology* 1984;152:273–277.

Calcified Fibrothorax

KEY FACTS

- Calcified fibrothorax, which is caused by calcification of dense fibrous tissue, can measure more than 2 cm in thickness.
- Calcified fibrothorax is most often the sequela of a prior exudative or hemorrhagic pleural effusion. Previous trauma with organization of hemothorax is another cause of calcified fibrothorax.
- Causes of massive unilateral calcified fibrothorax include tuberculous or other empyema.
- Asbestos-related pleural disease usually is bilateral and not diffusely calcified.
- Calcified fibrothorax can cause restrictive impairment of lung function.
- Radiographically, calcified pleural thickening is seen with contraction of the affected hemithorax. The pleural thickening is often greatest posterolaterally.
- Computed tomography scans show irregular pleural thickening composed of both soft tissue and calcified density. Both visceral and parietal pleural layers can be calcified.
- Most cases are incidental findings, but if severe ventilatory impairment occurs, surgical decortication is an option.

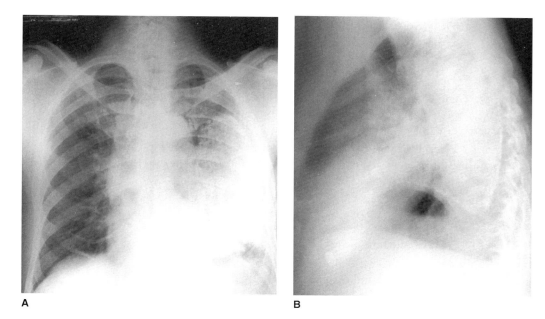

A   B

F I G U R E   2 2 - 2 2   Posteroanterior **(A)** and lateral **(B)** chest radiographs of a 69-year-old man who sustained a gunshot wound to the left chest 30 years prior show a large irregular dense opacity obscuring much of the left lung on the PA view and both lungs on the lateral view. On the lateral view, note the dense calcific opacity conforming to the outline of the pleural space.

Suggested Reading

Vix VA. Roentgenographic manifestations of pleural disease. *Semin Roentgenol* 1977;12: 277–286.

Asbestos-Related Pleural Disease

KEY FACTS

- Five asbestos-related pleural diseases are known: malignant mesothelioma and four benign pleural reactions—calcified or noncalcified pleural plaques, diffuse pleural thickening, rounded atelectasis, and pleural effusions.

- Pleural plaques occur in patients with occupational exposure to asbestos. Approximately 30 years from the time of first exposure to asbestos fibers is needed for a 50% chance of forming pleural plaques.

- These plaques usually involve the parietal pleura in typical locations: over the hemidiaphragms, in the posterior and paravertebral pleural surfaces in the lower thorax, and anterolateral pleural surfaces in the midthorax. Visceral pleural thickening is less common and is best seen in the pleural fissures. Pleural plaques are not predictive of asbestosis.

- Very small pleural plaques are usually not associated with clinically significant reductions in pulmonary function; however, the larger and more extensive the plaque formation, the more likely there is to be a component of restrictive pulmonary function, especially with diffuse pleural thickening.

- Diffuse pleural thickening appears as smooth, noninterrupted pleural opacity extending over at least one fourth of the chest wall. Diffuse pleural thickening is usually caused by the residua of a benign asbestos-related pleuritis with pleural effusion or confluent pleural plaques. Diffuse pleural thickening can be physiologically significant; it can cause restrictive pulmonary function. Associated pulmonary fibrosis is infrequent.

- Rounded atelectasis shows a typical wedge-shaped pleural-based pulmonary opacity with vessels sweeping into the center. Asbestos-related rounded atelectasis is a nonmalignant radiographic consequence of asbestos exposure that can mimic lung cancer. It occurs in the lung periphery, and is caused by pleural adhesions and fibrosis that deform the lung. Rounded atelectasis can occur after any insult that causes pleural scarring, including surgery or trauma, as well as asbestos-related pleural disease. Rounded atelectasis is usually a solitary finding, although it can be multiple. The posterior lung bases are the most common sites. With CT scanning, contiguity of the mass will always be seen with large, thick pleural plaques as a distinguishing, although not pathognomonic, feature. Sometimes it is impossible radiologically to distinguish rounded atelectasis from a lung cancer.

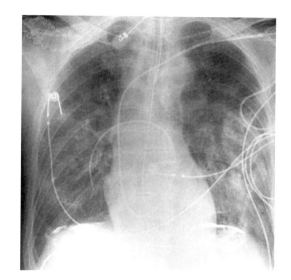

FIGURE 22-23

Anteroposterior chest radiograph of a 72-year-old man who worked for many years as a pipefitter shows typical asbestos-related calcified pleural plaques over both hemidiaphragms, and also seen as an irregular increase in density over the left midlung, as "en face" plaque. He is coincidentally intubated and catheterized for other medical reasons.

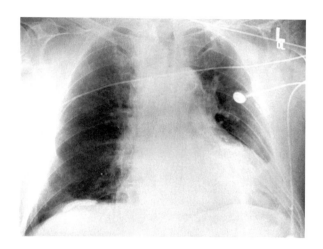

FIGURE 22-24

Posteroanterior chest radiograph of a 75-year-old man with a strong history of occupational asbestos exposure shows a thick asymmetric calcified pleural plaque on the right hemidiaphragm, as a somewhat atypical appearance.

(continued)

Asbestos-Related Pleural Disease (Continued)

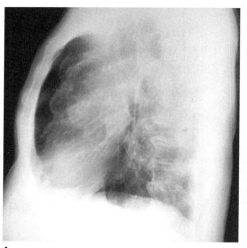
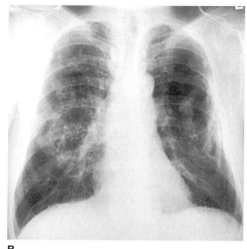

A   **B**

FIGURE 22-25   Posteroanterior **(A)** and lateral **(B)** chest radiographs of a 76-year-old man with significant exposure to asbestos clearly show, in both views, irregular opacities that overlay both lungs, representing calcified pleural plaques that have formed "en face" on the anterolateral pleural surfaces. In this case, only minimal plaque is seen on the hemidiaphragms.

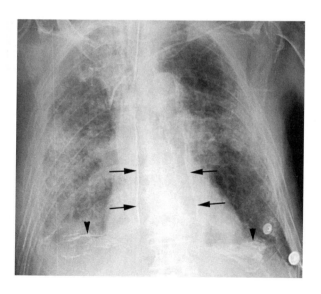

FIGURE 22-26

Anteroposterior chest radiograph of a 65-year-old man with a significant occupational exposure to asbestos shows typical calcified pleural plaques in the expected locations: "en face, along the spine (*arrows*), and over the hemidiaphragms (*arrowheads*). End-stage asbestosis is also noted. He is coincidentally intubated and catheterized for other medical reasons.

FIGURE 22-27

Computed tomography scan through the midchest of a 64-year-old man with a significant occupational exposure to asbestos shows a spectrum of different pleural plaques. Note the different thicknesses and different degrees of calcification that can be seen even in a single patient: calcified plaque (*arrows*), very thick calcified plaque (*double arrow*), and noncalcified plaque (*arrowhead*). The plaques occur in the typical locations: posteriorly and along the spine, and anterolaterally.

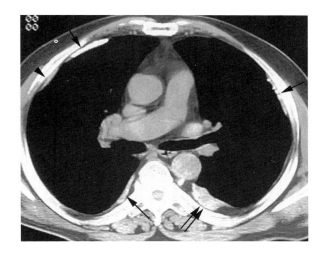

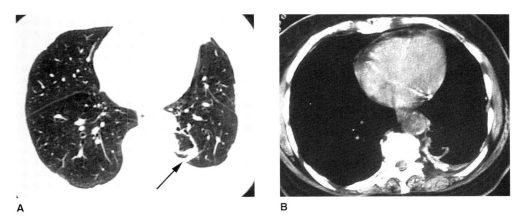

A   B

FIGURE 22-28   Computed tomography scan through the lower chest of a 74-year-old man with significant occupational exposure to asbestos shows an area of rounded atelectasis **(A)** (*arrow*) with a band of lung sweeping into a thick calcified pleural plaque **(B)**.

Suggested Reading

Gamsu G, Aberle DR, Lynch D. CT in the diagnosis of asbestos-related thoracic disease. *J Thorac Imaging* 1989;61–67.

Malignant Mesothelioma

KEY FACTS

- Malignant mesothelioma is more common in men aged more than 60 years. Presenting symptoms include nonpleuritic chest pain, shortness of breath, fever, sweats, weight loss, and fatigability.

- Up to 80% of cases are associated with asbestos exposure and the latency period usually exceeds 20 years. The size and shape of the asbestos fibers rather than the chemical composition are thought to affect carcinogenesis.

- Chest radiographs show evidence of asbestos exposure (e.g., pleural plaques) or the tumor itself with pleural thickening or associated pleural effusion.

- Computed tomography scans, which provide the best characterization and assessment of disease, can also show thickening or nodularity of the pleura, including the interlobar fissures. The tumor encases the lung in advanced cases. Calcified pleural plaques are seen in approximately 20% of patients, and effusions, which can be quite large, are seen in about 70% of patients.

- As malignant mesothelioma progresses, it invades locally to involve the esophagus, superior vena cava, vertebral bodies, nerves, ribs, mediastinum, and diaphragm. Fatigue and dyspnea result from arteriovenous shunting of blood in the trapped lung.

- Thoracentesis and pleural biopsy frequently do not provide adequate tissue sample to confirm the diagnosis. Thoracoscopy, however, can yield the diagnosis in most cases.

- The median duration of survival ranges from 4 to 18 months from the time of diagnosis.

- The differential diagnosis includes indolent pleural infections and metastatic pleural malignancy, usually an adenocarcinoma.

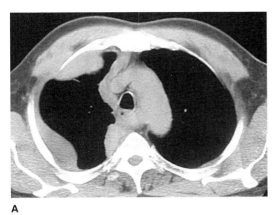
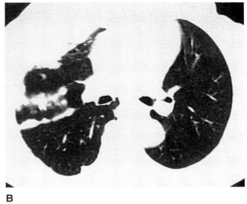

A   B

FIGURE 22-29   **(A, B)** Computed tomography scans through the chest of a 78-year-old man with significant occupational exposure to asbestos and malignant mesothelioma show a very thick, lobulated pleural mass that circumferentially nearly fills the pleural space. Note that the tumor extends, in a very lumpy fashion, into the major and minor fissures (lung window in **B**).

Suggested Reading

Kawashima A, Libshitz HI. Malignant pleural mesothelioma: CT manifestations in 50 cases. *AJR* 1990;155:965–969.

Pleural Fluid Versus Ascites

K E Y   F A C T S

- Pleural effusion in a subpulmonic location can be difficult to distinguish from ascites on cross-sectional imaging. If the diaphragm retains its normal curvature, a fluid collection located outside the diaphragm is pleural, whereas a collection within the diaphragm is intra-abdominal.

- On CT scans, the atelectatic inferior portion of the lower lobes can appear linear and mimic the diaphragm.

- Several signs have been described on CT to distinguish pleural fluid from ascites.

- The "bare" area of the liver abuts the posterior diaphragm. In patients with ascites, fluid cannot collect against the diaphragm, whereas pleural fluid can distribute along the entire length of the posterior hemidiaphragm.

- The interface sign refers to the greater haziness of the border between the fluid and adjacent liver or spleen in patients with pleural collections than those with ascites.

- The displaced crus sign denotes anterior displacement of the crus by pleural fluid, posterior displacement by ascites. This sign is considered less reliable than the other signs described.

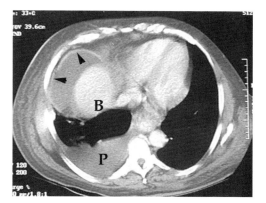

FIGURE 22-30

Computed tomography scan through the lower chest shows ascitic fluid within the normal curvature of the hemidiaphragm (*arrowheads*) and a fluid collection located posteriorly, outside the hemidiaphragm, which is pleural effusion (*P*). *B* denotes the bare area of the liver where peritoneal fluid cannot abut the posterior diaphragm.

Suggested Reading

Halvorsen RA, Fedyshin PJ, Korobkin M, et al. CT differentiation of pleural effusion from ascites: an evaluation of four signs using blinded analysis of 52 cases. *Invest Radiol* 1986; 21:391–395.

Localized Fibrous Tumor of Pleura

KEY FACTS

- Localized fibrous tumor of the pleura, formerly called "benign mesothelioma" is uncommon. Unlike malignant mesothelioma, no association with asbestos exposure is documented.
- The tumor is composed of mesenchymal cells that can undergo fibroblastic differentiation.
- Up to 80% of fibrous tumors originated from the visceral pleura. Most are benign but as many as 30% exhibit malignant behavior.
- Most patients are asymptomatic. Some have cough or chest pain. Fewer than 10% have hypertrophic osteoarthropathy or hypoglycemia.
- Radiographically, the tumor manifests as an oval or round well-defined lesion in contact with a pleural surface that can exceed 15 cm in diameter.
- The lesion can be subpleural or intrafissural. The tumor is pedunculated and may appear in different locations if patient position is altered.
- Computed tomography shows a well-marginated mass with acute angles to the pleural surface. Low attenuation can be present corresponding to necrosis. Substantial contrast enhancement is frequent and calcification occasionally occurs.

Suggested Reading
Ferretti GR, Chiles C, Choplin RH, et al. Localized benign fibrous tumors of the pleura. *AJR* 1997;169:683–686.

23   Diaphragm Abnormalities

Foramen of Morgagni Hernia

KEY FACTS

- Morgagni hernia is caused by abdominal viscera herniation between the sternal and costal attachments of the diaphragm.
- Morgagni hernia can occur at any age; it is most common on the right side.
- Most hernias are small and contain liver, omentum, or intestine.
- On chest radiographs, a Morgagni hernia appears as a mass in the right cardiophrenic angle.
- Air–fluid levels may be present if the hernia contains bowel.
- Computed tomography (CT) scans or magnetic resonance imaging (MRI) can show herniation of abdominal contents, and they can also exclude other possibilities including a pericardial cyst or an enlarged cardiac fat pad.

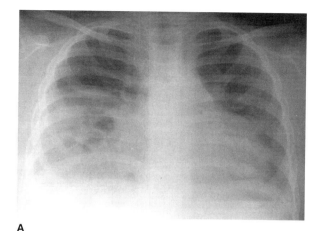

A

FIGURE 23-1

(**A**) Anteroposterior (AP) chest radiograph of a 5-year-old child shows an ill-defined increased opacity overlying the right lung base. A suggestion of loculated air is seen within the opacity, perhaps bowel loops. Frontal (**B**) and lateral (**C**) views of a barium enema show a loop of colon has herniated through a defect in the anterior (*arrow*) and medial portion of the right hemidiaphragm, typical for a foramen of Morgagni hernia.

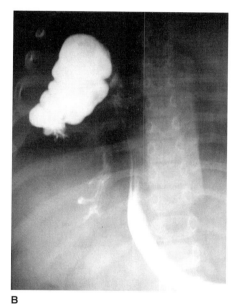

B

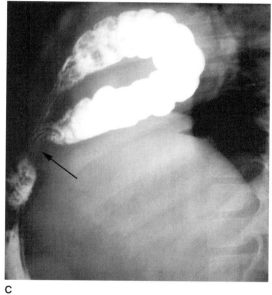

C

(continued)

Foramen of Morgagni Hernia (Continued)

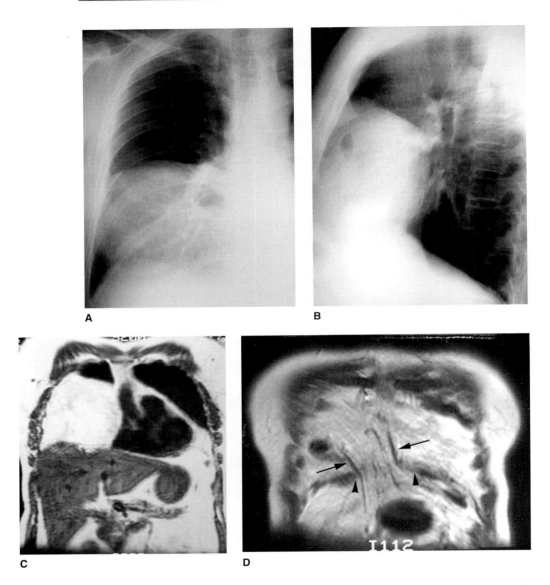

A   B

C   D

FIGURE 23-2   Posteroanterior (**A**) and lateral (**B**) chest radiographs of a 63-year-old asymptomatic man with a foramen of Morgagni hernia shows an ill-defined increased opacity overlying the right lung base, again with a loculated air collection suggestive of a loop of bowel. Coronal MRI shows the opacity is a collection of fat (**C**) that is extending into the right pleural space from the mesentery, through a defect (*arrowheads*) in the right hemidiaphragm (**D**). Note the mesenteric vessels coursing across the defect (*arrows*).

Suggested Reading

Paris F, Tarazona V, Casillas M. Hernia of Morgagni. *Thorax* 1973;28:631–636.

Foramen of Bochdalek Hernia

KEY FACTS

- Bochdalek hernia is caused by a failure of fusion, leaving a posterolateral diaphragmatic defect.

- Ninety percent of Bochdalek hernias are left-sided. However, Bochdalek hernias can be bilateral.

- Neonatal presentation with a Bochdalek-type hernia (congenital diaphragmatic hernia) can lead to severe respiratory compromise. The intestine, spleen, omentum, or kidney can herniate into the left chest.

- In older patients, the hernia is typically asymptomatic and is found incidentally.

- The adult type of hernia is far more common in the elderly and rarely is found in the young adult.

- On chest radiography, congenital hernia is recognized as loops of bowel in the left chest with contralateral shift of the mediastinum. A nasogastric tube tip may be identified in the left chest because of the upwardly displaced stomach.

- The chest radiograph in the adult type of Bochdalek hernia shows a posterior diaphragmatic convexity on the lateral view.

- Computed tomography scans in the adult patient with a Bochdalek hernia show the posterior defect in the diaphragm, which usually contains fat. Herniated spleen, kidney, or other abdominal viscera may be present.

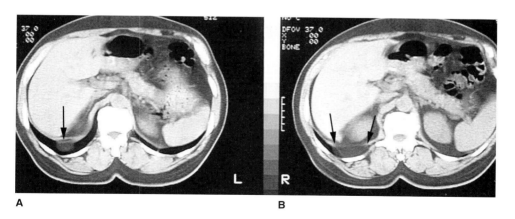

A   **B**

FIGURE 23-3   Computed tomography scan at the level of the diaphragm shows a small fat collection (*arrow* in **A**) on the posterior portion of the right hemidiaphragm, associated with a small defect in the hemidiaphragm (*arrows* in **B**), typical for a small, asymptomatic, incidental Bochdalek hernia.

Suggested Reading

Gale ME. Bochdalek hernia: prevalence and CT characteristics. *Radiology* 1985;156:449–452.

Diaphragmatic Eventration

KEY FACTS

- With an eventration, the diaphragm has areas of muscular thinning that have been replaced by a membranous sheet.
- Most commonly, the thinning involves one third to one half of the diaphragm, although the entire diaphragm can be affected.
- Total eventration most often involves the right hemidiaphragm and it is more common in women. Bilateral eventration is extremely rare.
- Nearly all patients with diaphragmatic eventration are asymptomatic.
- The diaphragmatic weakness in the areas of thinning allows upward bulging of the abdominal contents, although they do not extend through the diaphragm.
- On chest radiographs, the diaphragmatic bulging appears as a cephalad convexity of part or all of the affected diaphragm.
- On chest radiography, total eventration can mimic diaphragmatic hernia or elevation because of phrenic nerve paralysis.
- On fluoroscopy, the motion of the affected diaphragm in total eventration is poor or absent.

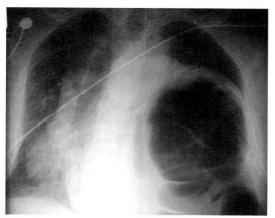

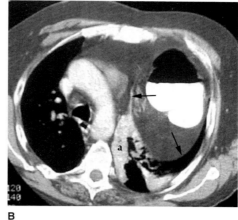

A   **B**

FIGURE 23-4   (**A**) Anteroposterior chest radiograph of a 75-year-old asymptomatic man shows a large air-filled and distended loop of colon apparently within the right pleural space. Note the shift of the mediastinum to the right. No history of trauma suggested a hemidiaphragm rupture. (**B**) CT scan at the level of the aortic arch shows normal mesenteric fat and a contrast and air filled loop of colon normally positioned below an elevated, thinned out left hemidiaphragm (*arrows*). Note the compressed, atelectatic left lower lobe (*a*).

Suggested Reading

Hesselink JR, Chung KJ, Peters ME, et al. Congenital partial eventration of the diaphragm. *Am J Roentgenol* 1978;131:417–419.

Traumatic Diaphragmatic Rupture

KEY FACTS

- Hemidiaphragm rupture can occur following both blunt and penetrating injuries. In blunt injury, high intra-abdominal pressures are speculated as the usual mechanism of hemidiaphragm rupture, although penetrating rib fractures can also lacerate the hemidiaphragm.

- Incidence of right-sided versus left-sided hemidiaphragm rupture after blunt abdominal trauma is controversial. The classic teaching is that 90% of ruptures are left-sided; however, the true incidence may be more equal, the liver just prevents clinical manifestations.

- Of clinically significant hemidiaphragm ruptures, 90% are overlooked initially and 90% of strangulated diaphragmatic hernias occur from trauma.

- Hemidiaphragm rupture can occur in the acute trauma setting or be delayed by days, weeks, or even years.

- Hemidiaphragm rupture is associated with other significant intra-abdominal injuries in most cases.

- Small lacerations of the hemidiaphragm are difficult to detect; the chest radiograph can be normal.

- With a large hemidiaphragm rupture, chest radiographs are never normal. Radiographic findings of left hemidiaphragm rupture include:

    Loops of bowel, usually stomach and colon, within the thorax

    Nasogastric tube showing the position of the stomach within the thorax

    Left pleural effusion

    Ill-defined soft-tissue mass obscuring the left hemidiaphragm

    Left basilar lung atelectasis

- Radiographic findings of right hemidiaphragm rupture include:

    Apparent elevation of the hemidiaphragm

    Pleural effusion

    Rarely, loops of bowel or the entire liver within the thorax (must be a very large laceration)

- Computed tomography and MRI scans can be used as adjunctive diagnostic tests in difficult cases, especially using coronal imaging planes.

FIGURE 23-5

Coronal reformatted, contrast-enhanced CT scan through the lower chest of a 32-year-old man who suffered a motor-vehicle accident 5 days earlier shows a "mushroom" of normally enhancing liver (*L*) extending above the expected position of the right hemidiaphragm (*arrows*), in this case a delayed traumatic rupture of the diaphragm.

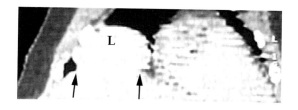

Suggested Reading

Gelman R, Mirvis SE, Gens D. Diaphragmatic rupture due to blunt trauma: sensitivity of plain chest radiographs. *AJR* 1991;156:51–57.

COMMON MEDICAL PROBLEMS

24 Common Medical Problems

Asthma

KEY FACTS

- Asthma is episodic, nonspecific hyper-reactivity of the lower airways that leads to reversible small airways obstruction.
- Asthma is very common, occurring in up to 5% of adults and 10% of children.
- The chest radiograph can be normal, but nonspecific findings include:
  Hyperinflation
  Hypoinflation with multiple focal areas of atelectasis distal to the obstructed airways
  Pneumomediastinum
  Interstitial pulmonary emphysema
  Complicating pneumonia
- "All that wheezes is not asthma." Other causes to consider include:
  Congestive heart failure
  Bronchitis and emphysema
  Airway tumor or foreign body
  Recurrent pulmonary emboli

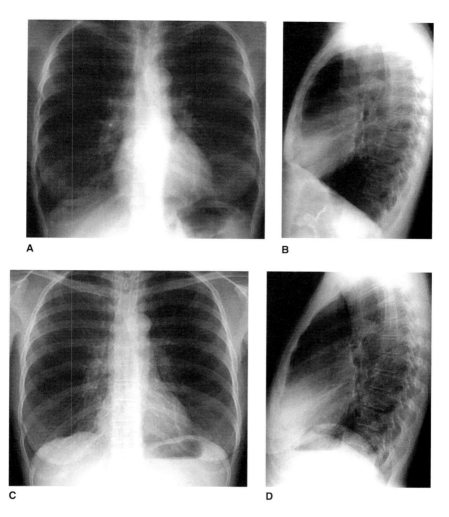

F I G U R E   2 4 - 1   Two sets of posteroanterior and lateral radiographs of a 38-year-old woman with asthma obtained during **(A, B)** and after **(C, D)** an asthma attack. Note that the hyperinflation, with increased lucency of the lungs and flattened hemidiaphragms, resolves after bronchodilator therapy.

Suggested Reading

Clausen JL. The diagnosis of emphysema, chronic bronchitis, and asthma. *Clin Chest Med* 1990;11:405–416.

Chest Pain

KEY FACTS

- In the nontrauma setting, many causes of chest pain can be potentially life threatening, such as:

  Angina pectoris and myocardial infarction

  Pneumonia

  Aortic dissection

  Spontaneous pneumothorax

  Pulmonary embolism

  Pericarditis

- Other less serious causes of chest pain include:

  Costochondritis, muscle strain, and arthritis

  Pneumonia and bronchitis

  Rib fracture

  Esophageal disease

  Referred pain from the cervical spine or abdomen

  Herpes zoster

- Chest radiographs can often suggest a specific cause, such as congestive heart failure, pneumonia, wide mediastinum, rib fracture, or pneumothorax.

- Although the chest radiograph is often sufficient to suggest a diagnosis, it should also be considered a screening tool to suggest, by either absence or presence of findings, other diagnostic tests (e.g., chest computed tomography [CT] or magnetic resonance imaging [MRI] scan for aortic dissection, ventilation–perfusion scan for pulmonary embolism, coronary arteriography for coronary artery disease, or echocardiography for pericardial disease).

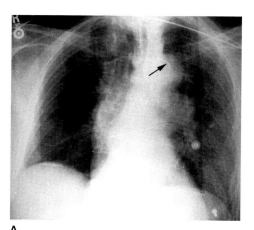

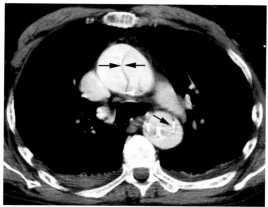

A   B

F I G U R E   2 4 - 2   (**A**) Anteroposterior chest radiograph of a 78-year-old man with stabbing chest pain radiating to the back shows apparent medial displacement of a rim of calcification in the aortic arch (*arrow*). This sign is suggestive of aortic dissection, especially when it is a new finding when compared with prior radiographs, and more than 7 mm of intimal calcification displacement is seen. (**B**) Contrast-enhanced CT scan of the chest from the same patient shows a typical aortic dissection with an intimal flap separating the true and false lumens (*face-to-face arrows*). Note the calcified intima displacement, which corresponds to the chest radiographic finding (*arrow*).

Suggested Reading

Godwin JD. Conventional CT of the aorta. *J Thorac Imaging* 1990;5:18–31.

Cough

KEY FACTS

- Cough in the acute setting most commonly results from inflammatory or mechanical causes; exposure to extremely cold air or chemicals are less common causes. Neoplastic disease of the airways or lung (benign or malignant) is another important cause.

- Inflammatory causes of cough secondary to a variety of infectious agents include laryngitis, tracheitis, bronchitis, and pneumonia. Also consider noninfectious causes such as airway edema or spasm (asthma).

- Mechanical causes of cough include foreign body aspiration, especially in children, dust exposures, and neoplastic disease.

- Chemical causes of cough include cigarette smoking and smoke inhalation.

- Chest radiographs are helpful, although it depends on the cause of the cough; they directly show lung or airway neoplasms, or pneumonia. The chest radiograph can also show more subtle abnormalities such as nonspecific central bronchial wall thickening in smoke inhalation, bronchitis, or asthma.

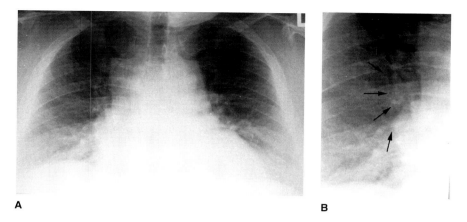

A   **B**

FIGURE 24-3   Posteroanterior **(A)** chest radiograph and close-up **(B)** of the right hilum of a 34
year-old-man with chronic cough show low lung volumes and peribronchial thick-
ening (cuffing) consistent with the clinical diagnosis of bronchitis (*arrows*).

Suggested Reading

Clausen JL. The diagnosis of emphysema, chronic bronchitis, and asthma. *Clin Chest Med*
1990;11:405–416.

Dysphagia

KEY FACTS

- Dysphagia, which is difficulty swallowing, is related to either oropharyngeal disease or esophageal disease. The sensation is usually referred to the suprasternal notch.

- Chronic dysphagia is usually caused by a prior insult to the esophagus such as a peptic or lye stricture, a Schatzki's ring, or carcinoma. Less commonly the cause is scleroderma or achalasia.

- Acute dysphagia is more likely to represent an emetic injury such as Boerhaave's syndrome, or swallowing of a foreign body, such as a coin, large piece of meat, or fish bone. An acute presentation of the above chronic causes should always be considered.

- In the acute setting, the chest radiograph can show most radiopaque foreign bodies. Esophageal rupture (Boerhaave's syndrome) will usually show pneumomediastinum and left pleural fluid collection (containing gastric contents) (see Chap. 17).

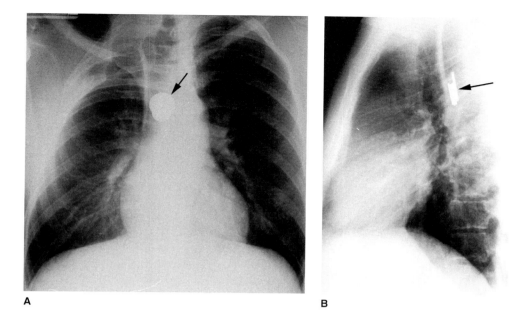

A
B

FIGURE 24-4   Posteroanterior **(A)** and lateral **(B)** chest radiographs of a 20-year-old-man with a psychiatric disturbance, complaining of difficulty swallowing, show several coins (*arrows*) lodged in the midesophagus. Note the mild distention of the proximal esophagus.

Suggested Reading
Levine MS, Rubesin SE. Radiologic investigation of dysphagia. *AJR* 1990;154:1157–1163.

Dyspnea

KEY FACTS

- Dyspnea is an abnormal, uncomfortable awareness of breathing with varying degrees of exertion.
- Common causes of dyspnea include:

  Diffuse lung diseases such as pulmonary fibrosis and severe pneumonia

  Obstructive airways diseases such as emphysema and asthma, and mechanical obstructions such as lung cancer or foreign body

  Heart diseases such as ischemic cardiomyopathy with congestive left-side heart failure

  Pleural processes such as pneumothorax or pleural effusions

  Acute and chronic pulmonary thromboembolic disease

  Chest wall or respiratory muscle diseases such as phrenic nerve injury, kyphoscoliosis, and muscular dystrophy
- Chest radiographs are helpful in distinguishing many of these causes.
- Chest CT scanning (especially high resolution CT) is most helpful in evaluating diffuse infiltrative and obstructive lung diseases and neoplastic disease.

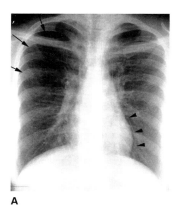 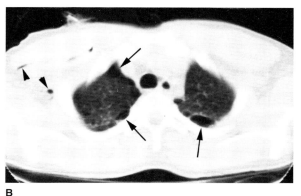

A   B

FIGURE 24-5   (A) Posteroanterior chest radiograph of a 40-year-old-man with sudden onset of dyspnea (no history of trauma) shows a large pneumothorax (*arrows*), in this case, spontaneous, and a pneumomediastinum (*arrowheads*). (B) CT scan through the lung apices in this patient, after the pneumothorax was successfully treated, shows multiple apical bullae (*arrows*), presumably the cause of the spontaneous pneumothorax, and residual subcutaneous emphysema (*arrowheads*).

Suggested Reading

Lesur O, Delorme N, Fromaget JM, et al. Computed tomography in the etiologic assessment of idiopathic spontaneous pneumothorax. *Chest* 1990;98:341–347.

Hemoptysis

KEY FACTS

- The causes of expectorated blood or blood-stained sputum—hemoptysis—are very similar to cough; the most common being bronchitis, bronchiectasis, and pyogenic pneumonia (especially *Klebsiella*).

- Other less common causes include lung cancer, pulmonary thromboembolic disease, pulmonary contusions or lacerations, and congestive heart failure. Pulmonary hemorrhage syndromes and bleeding diastheses are rare causes.

- The cause of hemoptysis can remain undiscovered in up to 15% of patients.

- It is important to determine the origin of bleeding, as this can direct further diagnostic and therapeutic procedures such as bronchial artery embolization or bronchoscopy.

- The chest radiograph is essential in patients with hemoptysis; it can usually distinguish the more common causes such as pneumonia, heart failure, and neoplastic disease. Because chest CT scanning is very sensitive in identifying the central lung cancers and in diagnosing bronchiectasis, it should usually be obtained prior to bronchoscopy in all patients presenting with hemoptysis.

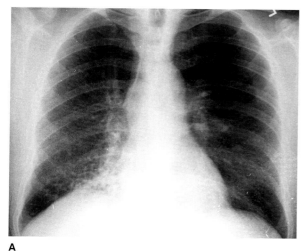

A

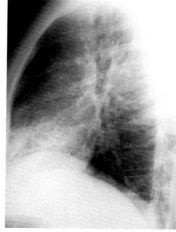

B

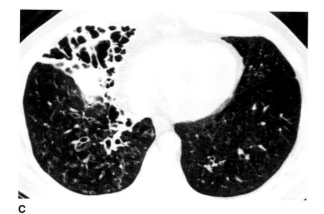

C

FIGURE 24-6

(**A, B**) Posteroanterior and lateral chest radiographs of a 37-year-old-man with a history of chronic sputum production and recent onset of hemoptysis show multiple ring-shaped opacities in the distribution of the right middle lobe suggestive of bronchiectasis. (**C**) Chest CT scan through the middle lobe confirms extensive cystic bronchiectasis as the cause of hemoptysis. Milder, cylindrical bronchiectasis is seen in the right lower lobe as well.

Suggested Reading

McGuinness G, Beacher JR, Harkin TJ, et al. Hemoptysis: prospective high-resolution CT/bronchoscopic correlation. *Chest* 1994;105:1155–1162.

Subject Index